AF446428

Community Health Worker

-

The Comprehensive Guide

by

VIRUTI SHIVAN

Masters in Clinical Psychology (Major)

"In books, as in life, it's not the size or looks but the content that matters."

DISCLAIMER: The information in this book is provided for general informational purposes only and is not intended as professional advice. Although every effort has been made to ensure the accuracy and completeness of the information, the author and publisher do not assume responsibility for errors, inaccuracies, omissions, inconsistencies, or the impact of future advancements or updates in technology and information. This book is not a substitute for proper training, diagnosis, treatment, or guidance from qualified professionals. Readers are encouraged to consult experts in the relevant fields and independently verify the information when necessary. Any slights of people, places, or organizations are unintentional and purely coincidental.

Introduction

Welcome to "Community Health Worker - The Comprehensive Guide," a pivotal resource designed to empower and enlighten those at the forefront of community health. This book is a tribute to the resilience, dedication, and impact of Community Health Workers (CHWs) worldwide. It serves as a beacon for aspiring and seasoned CHWs alike, offering a comprehensive toolkit to navigate the multifaceted landscape of global health delivery.

As we embark on this journey together, the chapters ahead are structured to provide a deep dive into the essential skills, knowledge, and strategies that define successful community health initiatives. From understanding the foundational aspects of public health to mastering complex interventions for disease prevention and health promotion, our aim is to enhance the effectiveness and reach of CHWs in their communities.

This guide is meticulously crafted to ensure readability and practical application, with each chapter including real-life scenarios, personal anecdotes, and hypothetical situations that offer a window into the challenges and triumphs faced by CHWs. Exercises at the end of each chapter are designed to test knowledge and reinforce learning, ensuring that readers not only absorb the information but are also able to apply it in their work.

In the absence of images or illustrations, we rely on vivid storytelling and practical examples to paint a comprehensive picture of the role of CHWs. This approach allows us to sidestep potential copyright issues while focusing on delivering engaging and informative content that resonates with our readers.

As you turn the pages of this guide, remember that the journey of a thousand miles begins with a single step. Let this book be your first step toward making a lasting impact in the field of community health.

Chapter 1: Understanding Community Health

1.1 The Role of Community Health Workers

Community Health Workers (CHWs) are the linchpins in the wheel of healthcare delivery within communities, especially in areas where access to formal healthcare systems is limited or non-existent. Their role transcends the boundaries of mere health facilitators to become advocates, educators, and liaisons between healthcare systems and communities. This subchapter delves into the multifaceted roles of CHWs, shedding light on how they are pivotal in fostering healthier communities through a grassroots approach.

CHWs serve as the first point of contact in their communities for health-related concerns, providing critical services such as basic health screenings, health education, and referrals to medical professionals when necessary. They are uniquely positioned to effect change due to their understanding of the cultural and social nuances of the communities they serve. This deep-rooted connection enables CHWs to communicate effectively, promoting health practices that are culturally sensitive and more likely to be accepted and sustained within the community.

Moreover, CHWs play a vital role in preventive health care. By educating community members on health promotion and disease prevention strategies, they empower individuals to take charge of their health. This education covers a broad range of topics, from nutrition and exercise to the importance of regular health check-ups and vaccinations. Through these efforts, CHWs contribute significantly to the reduction of health disparities and the burden on secondary and tertiary healthcare services.

In addition to preventive care, CHWs are instrumental in managing and mitigating health crises within communities. They are often on the front lines during outbreaks of communicable diseases, where they assist in disease surveillance, provide critical information on disease prevention, and support the community's emergency response efforts. Their ability to quickly mobilize and address health concerns is crucial in preventing the spread of diseases and minimizing health impacts on the community.

The effectiveness of a CHW lies in their approach to health as a holistic concept, recognizing that health outcomes are influenced by a wide array of factors including socioeconomic status, education, environment, and access to healthcare services. By addressing these determinants of health, CHWs contribute to the creation of environments that promote well-being and prevent illness.

Exercise: 10 MCQs with Answers at the End

This section will test your understanding of the role of Community Health Workers in improving community health. The questions cover various aspects of CHWs' responsibilities, including health promotion, disease prevention, and their role in emergency responses. Answers are provided at the end of the chapter to help you assess your grasp of the material discussed.

1.2 Principles of Community Health

Community health is grounded in several core principles that guide the work of healthcare professionals, including Community Health Workers (CHWs), in their efforts to improve the health and well-being of communities. Understanding these principles is crucial for anyone involved in community health as they form the foundation for effective health promotion and disease prevention strategies. This subchapter explores these essential principles, emphasizing their importance in shaping the approaches and interventions employed in community health.

Equity and Access to Healthcare

At the heart of community health is the principle of equity and the commitment to ensuring all community members have equal access to healthcare services, regardless of socioeconomic status, gender, ethnicity, or geographical location. This principle challenges health disparities and aims to eliminate barriers to healthcare access, including financial, cultural, and linguistic barriers, thereby promoting a more inclusive health system.

Prevention Over Cure

A proactive approach to health, focusing on prevention rather than cure, is a fundamental principle of community health. By emphasizing preventive measures such as vaccinations, health education, and lifestyle modifications, community health initiatives aim to reduce the incidence of chronic diseases and avoidable healthcare issues. This principle not only leads to healthier communities but also reduces the economic burden on healthcare systems.

Community Participation and Empowerment

Community health is most effective when the community members themselves are involved in the planning, implementation, and evaluation of health programs. This participatory approach ensures that health interventions are tailored to the unique needs and preferences of the community, thereby increasing their relevance and effectiveness. Empowering communities to take charge of their health also fosters a sense of ownership and responsibility towards improving health outcomes.

Intersectoral Collaboration

Recognizing that health is influenced by a wide range of factors beyond the healthcare sector, community health emphasizes the importance of intersectoral collaboration. Partnerships with sectors such as education, housing, environment, and transportation are vital to address the social determinants of health and create supportive environments that promote well-being.

Sustainability

Sustainability in community health involves developing interventions that are not only effective in the short term but also maintainable over the long term. This requires building the capacity of local health systems and communities, ensuring the availability of resources, and fostering resilient structures that can adapt to changing health needs and challenges.

Holistic Health

Community health adopts a holistic view of health, recognizing that physical, mental, social, and environmental health are interconnected. This approach advocates for comprehensive health strategies that address the full spectrum of health needs, promoting overall well-being rather than focusing narrowly on specific diseases or conditions.

Understanding and applying these principles of community health is essential for CHWs and all health professionals working at the community level. By integrating these principles into their work, they can more effectively contribute to the development of healthy, resilient, and equitable communities.

1.3 Challenges in Community Health Delivery

The journey towards achieving optimal community health is fraught with numerous challenges that can impede the delivery of effective healthcare services. These challenges range from systemic issues to more localized problems, each requiring a unique approach and solution. Understanding these obstacles is crucial for Community Health Workers (CHWs) and other health professionals as it prepares them to navigate these difficulties with resilience and innovation. This subchapter identifies and explores the significant challenges in community health delivery, providing a comprehensive overview that underscores the complexities of healthcare provision at the community level.

Limited Resources and Infrastructure

One of the most significant barriers to effective community health delivery is the scarcity of resources and inadequate infrastructure, especially in low-income communities and developing countries. This scarcity encompasses a broad range of issues, including limited access to medical supplies, insufficient healthcare facilities, and a shortage of trained healthcare personnel. Such constraints not only limit the availability of health services but also impact the quality of care that communities receive.

Cultural and Language Barriers

Cultural beliefs and language differences can significantly affect health delivery and outcomes. Misunderstandings or miscommunications between healthcare providers and community members can lead to mistrust, reduced compliance with medical advice, and lower uptake of health services. Additionally, certain cultural beliefs may discourage the use of formal healthcare services, leading to delays in seeking necessary medical attention.

Health Literacy

Health literacy, or the ability to obtain, process, and understand basic health information and services needed to make appropriate health decisions, is a critical challenge. Low health literacy levels can hinder the effectiveness of health education and promotion efforts, leading to poorer health outcomes and increased health disparities.

Environmental and Social Determinants of Health

The environment in which people live and work significantly influences their health outcomes. Issues such as pollution, inadequate housing, lack of clean water and sanitation, and social determinants like poverty, education, and unemployment can create or exacerbate health problems. Addressing these determinants requires a multi-sectoral approach that goes beyond the healthcare system.

Non-Communicable Diseases (NCDs)

The rise of non-communicable diseases (NCDs) such as diabetes, cardiovascular diseases, and cancer poses a growing challenge for community health. These conditions require long-term management and care, putting additional strain on already limited community health resources and requiring innovative strategies for prevention, management, and treatment.

Access to Healthcare Services

Even when healthcare services are available, accessing them can be a challenge for many community members due to factors such as distance, cost, and lack of transportation. These barriers can lead to significant delays in receiving care, exacerbating health conditions and leading to preventable complications.

Data Collection and Monitoring

Effective community health delivery relies on accurate and timely health data to inform decision-making and resource allocation. However, challenges in data collection, including lack of standardized tools, inadequate training, and resource constraints, can hinder the monitoring and evaluation of health interventions.

Addressing these challenges requires a concerted effort from all stakeholders, including governments, healthcare providers, communities, and international organizations. By understanding and tackling these obstacles, CHWs and other health professionals can better serve their communities, improving health outcomes and enhancing the quality of life for individuals across the globe.

1.4 Exercise: 10 MCQs with Answers at the End

This exercise is designed to test your understanding of the topics covered in Chapter 1: Understanding Community Health. Each question focuses on a key aspect discussed in the subchapters, including the role of Community Health Workers, principles of community health, and challenges in community health delivery. Answers are provided at the end to help you assess your comprehension and reinforce your learning.

Multiple Choice Questions

1. What is a primary role of Community Health Workers (CHWs)?

   A) Provide advanced medical care

   B) Conduct major surgical operations

   C) Act as liaisons between communities and the healthcare system

   D) Design healthcare policies

2. Which principle emphasizes the importance of involving community members in the health program planning process?

   A) Equity and Access to Healthcare

   B) Prevention Over Cure

   C) Community Participation and Empowerment

D) Intersectoral Collaboration

3. A major barrier to effective community health delivery is:

A) Excessive healthcare facilities

B) High levels of health literacy

C) Limited resources and infrastructure

D) Overabundance of medical supplies

4. Which of the following is NOT a focus of community health?

A) Treating non-communicable diseases

B) Addressing cultural and language barriers

C) Ignoring social determinants of health

D) Promoting preventive health measures

5. The principle of ______________ focuses on taking proactive measures to prevent health issues rather than treating them after they arise.

A) Sustainability

B) Prevention Over Cure

C) Holistic Health

D) Equity and Access to Healthcare

6. Cultural beliefs and language differences can lead to:

A) Improved compliance with medical advice

B) Higher uptake of health services

C) Misunderstandings between healthcare providers and community members

D) Excessive trust in healthcare systems

7. Health literacy is crucial for:

A) Increasing the complexity of healthcare information

B) Making inappropriate health decisions

C) Understanding basic health information and services

D) Reducing communication between CHWs and community members

8. Environmental and social determinants of health include all EXCEPT:

A) Education level

B) Pollution

C) Access to medical supplies

D) Employment status

9. Non-communicable diseases (NCDs) are a challenge for community health because:

A) They do not affect communities

B) They require no long-term management

C) They put a strain on limited resources

D) They are easily preventable with minimal effort

10. Effective community health delivery relies on:

A) Ignoring cultural and language barriers

B) Limited participation of community members

C) Accurate and timely health data

D) Sole focus on treatment rather than prevention

Answers

1. C) Act as liaisons between communities and the healthcare system

2. C) Community Participation and Empowerment

3. C) Limited resources and infrastructure

4. C) Ignoring social determinants of health

5. B) Prevention Over Cure

6. C) Misunderstandings between healthcare providers and community members

7. C) Understanding basic health information and services

8. C) Access to medical supplies

9. C) They put a strain on limited resources

10. C) Accurate and timely health data

Chapter 2: Health Promotion and Disease Prevention

2.1 Strategies for Health Promotion

Health promotion involves empowering individuals and communities to increase control over their health, resulting in an improvement of their overall well-being. This proactive approach to health encourages people to adopt healthy behaviors and make changes that reduce the risk of developing chronic diseases and other health conditions. This subchapter outlines effective strategies for health promotion, highlighting how these approaches can be integrated into community health initiatives to foster a culture of health.

Educational Programs

One of the cornerstone strategies for health promotion is the development and implementation of educational programs. These programs aim to raise awareness about healthy behaviors, such as nutrition, physical activity, and the importance of regular health screenings. By providing individuals with knowledge about how their lifestyle choices can impact their health, educational programs empower them to make informed decisions that promote their well-being.

Community Engagement

Engaging the community in health promotion activities is critical for ensuring that these initiatives are relevant, accessible, and sustainable. This can involve organizing health fairs, workshops, and support groups that address specific health concerns within the community. By involving community members in the planning and execution of these activities, health promoters can ensure that the interventions are tailored to the unique needs and preferences of the community.

Policy Advocacy

Advocating for policies that create healthier environments is another vital strategy for health promotion. This can include efforts to regulate tobacco use, improve food and water quality, and promote physical activity through the development of parks and recreational facilities. Policy changes can provide a supportive environment that makes it easier for individuals to adopt and maintain healthy behaviors.

Technology and Social Media

The use of technology and social media has emerged as a powerful tool in health promotion. Digital platforms can be used to disseminate health information widely and quickly, engage with individuals directly, and provide support and motivation for adopting healthier lifestyles. Apps, websites, and social media can also be utilized to track health behaviors, provide personalized feedback, and connect individuals with similar health goals.

Collaborations with Healthcare Providers

Collaborating with healthcare providers to integrate health promotion activities into routine care can significantly enhance the impact of these initiatives. Healthcare providers can play a crucial role in identifying at-risk individuals, delivering personalized health promotion messages, and referring patients to community resources that support healthy living.

Environmental Changes

Making changes to the physical and social environment can significantly influence health behaviors. This strategy focuses on creating environments that support health, such as safe spaces for physical activity, access to healthy foods, and reducing exposure to harmful substances. Environmental changes can help make the healthy choice the easy choice for individuals.

Effective health promotion requires a multifaceted approach that combines individual, community, and policy-level interventions. By employing a combination of these strategies, community health workers and health promoters can work towards creating communities where healthy choices are accessible, encouraged, and supported.

2.2 Preventing Communicable Diseases

Preventing communicable diseases within communities is a critical aspect of public health that requires comprehensive strategies and coordinated efforts. Communicable diseases, also known as infectious or transmissible diseases, can spread from person to person or through vectors, making their prevention a cornerstone of community health efforts. This subchapter focuses on key strategies for preventing the spread of communicable diseases, emphasizing the role of community health workers (CHWs) in implementing these strategies effectively.

Vaccination Programs

Vaccination is one of the most effective means of preventing communicable diseases. Implementing vaccination programs that ensure high coverage in the community can protect against a wide range of infectious diseases, including measles, polio, and influenza. CHWs play a pivotal role in these programs by educating the community about the benefits of vaccination, identifying unvaccinated individuals, and facilitating access to vaccination services.

Health Education and Awareness Campaigns

Raising awareness about communicable diseases and how they are transmitted is essential for prevention. Health education campaigns can inform community members about the importance of personal hygiene practices, such as regular handwashing with soap and water, covering the mouth and nose when coughing or sneezing, and safe food preparation methods. CHWs can deliver these messages through community meetings, schools, and door-to-door visits, tailoring the information to the cultural and social context of the community.

Safe Water, Sanitation, and Hygiene (WASH) Practices

Access to safe water, adequate sanitation, and good hygiene practices is fundamental in preventing the spread of waterborne and foodborne diseases. CHWs can advocate for improvements in water and sanitation infrastructure, conduct hygiene education sessions, and distribute hygiene kits to promote healthy practices.

Disease Surveillance and Reporting

Effective disease surveillance systems are crucial for the early detection of communicable disease outbreaks. CHWs can contribute to surveillance efforts by monitoring health trends within the community, reporting unusual patterns of illness, and collaborating with health authorities to investigate and respond to potential outbreaks.

Isolation and Quarantine Measures

In the event of an outbreak, isolating individuals with communicable diseases and quarantining those who have been exposed can help prevent further transmission. CHWs can support these measures by educating the community about the importance of isolation and quarantine, assisting with the implementation of these measures, and providing support to affected individuals and families.

Vector Control

For diseases transmitted by vectors, such as mosquitoes, flies, and ticks, controlling the vector population can significantly reduce disease transmission. CHWs can participate in vector control activities, such as distributing insecticide-treated bed nets, eliminating standing water where mosquitoes breed, and educating the community about the use of repellents and protective clothing.

Preventing communicable diseases is a complex task that requires the active involvement of the entire community, supported by a strong public health infrastructure. Through a combination of vaccination, education, sanitation, surveillance, isolation, and vector control strategies, communities can significantly reduce the burden of communicable diseases.

2.3 Non-Communicable Diseases: Prevention and Care

Non-Communicable Diseases (NCDs), such as cardiovascular diseases, cancers, chronic respiratory diseases, and diabetes, pose a significant public health challenge globally. Unlike communicable diseases, NCDs are not passed from person to person but are caused by a combination of genetic, physiological, environmental, and behavioral factors. Preventing and managing these diseases requires a comprehensive and sustained effort, focusing on both individual and community-wide interventions. This subchapter explores effective strategies for the prevention and care of NCDs, highlighting the crucial role of Community Health Workers (CHWs) in these efforts.

Lifestyle Modifications for Prevention

Preventing NCDs often starts with lifestyle modifications aimed at reducing risk factors. Key interventions include promoting a healthy diet, increasing physical activity, avoiding tobacco use, and reducing alcohol consumption. CHWs can lead by example and educate the community on making healthier lifestyle choices, organizing group activities that encourage physical exercise, and offering nutrition workshops to share knowledge on balanced diets.

Screening and Early Detection

Early detection of NCDs through regular screening can significantly improve outcomes by facilitating early intervention and treatment. CHWs can play a vital role in raising awareness about the importance of screening and guiding community members on when and where to access these services. For conditions like hypertension and diabetes, CHWs can also be trained to perform basic screenings and refer individuals with abnormal results to healthcare facilities for further evaluation.

Management and Care

Effective management of NCDs often requires a coordinated care approach that includes medication management, regular monitoring of symptoms, lifestyle adjustments, and psychological support. CHWs can assist in this process by providing education on disease management, reminding patients about medication schedules, and offering support for lifestyle changes. Moreover, they can act as a bridge between patients and healthcare providers, ensuring that individuals living with NCDs receive comprehensive care that is tailored to their needs.

Mental Health Support

The psychological impact of living with NCDs cannot be underestimated. Mental health support is a critical component of NCD care, as conditions like depression and anxiety can coexist with physical health issues, affecting patients' quality of life and treatment outcomes. CHWs can offer emotional support, facilitate support groups, and refer individuals to mental health services when necessary.

Community-Based Interventions

Addressing the broader determinants of NCDs requires community-based interventions that target the environmental and social factors contributing to these diseases. Initiatives such as creating smoke-free zones, promoting safe and accessible physical activity spaces, and advocating for healthy food options in schools and workplaces can help reduce the prevalence of NCD risk factors in the community.

Palliative Care

For individuals with advanced NCDs, palliative care becomes an essential component of the care continuum. CHWs can provide palliative support by offering comfort care, educating families on pain management, and ensuring that patients live their final days with dignity.

Preventing and managing NCDs is a multifaceted challenge that requires ongoing education, support, and care coordination. CHWs, with their unique position within the community, are instrumental in implementing strategies that can significantly impact the prevention and management of these diseases, improving the overall health and well-being of the community.

2.4 Exercise: 10 MCQs with Answers at the End

This section contains multiple-choice questions designed to test your understanding of the concepts discussed in Chapter 2: Health Promotion and Disease Prevention. The questions cover strategies for health promotion, preventing communicable diseases, non-communicable diseases prevention and care, and the roles of Community Health Workers (CHWs) in these processes. Review the questions carefully and choose the best answer for each. Answers are provided at the end to help you assess your knowledge and understanding of the topics covered.

Multiple Choice Questions

1. Which of the following is an effective strategy for health promotion?

   A) Decreasing physical activity

   B) Increasing tobacco use

   C) Promoting a healthy diet

   D) Encouraging excessive alcohol consumption

2. The primary role of vaccination programs in preventing communicable diseases is to:

   A) Reduce the efficacy of antibiotics

   B) Increase the number of people susceptible to infectious diseases

   C) Provide immunity against specific infections

   D) Promote the spread of viral diseases

3. A key component of preventing non-communicable diseases (NCDs) is:

   A) Avoiding regular health screenings

   B) Increasing sedentary lifestyle choices

   C) Promoting physical activity

   D) Encouraging high intake of processed foods

4. Community Health Workers (CHWs) contribute to disease surveillance by:

   A) Ignoring unusual patterns of illness

   B) Reporting unusual patterns of illness to health authorities

   C) Discouraging community members from seeking medical advice

   D) Increasing the spread of communicable diseases

5. Which of the following is NOT a benefit of community engagement in health promotion activities?

   A) Tailored health interventions

   B) Reduced relevance of health initiatives

   C) Increased accessibility of health services

   D) Enhanced sustainability of health programs

6. Early detection of non-communicable diseases (NCDs) can be facilitated by:

   A) Regular screening and early intervention

   B) Ignoring symptoms of chronic diseases

   C) Delaying treatment until diseases progress

   D) Discouraging the use of healthcare services

7. Safe Water, Sanitation, and Hygiene (WASH) practices prevent the spread of:

   A) Non-communicable diseases

   B) Waterborne and foodborne diseases

   C) Physical inactivity

   D) Genetic disorders

8. Mental health support for individuals with NCDs is important because:

   A) It worsens the physical symptoms of NCDs

   B) Psychological conditions do not affect individuals with NCDs

   C) It can improve treatment outcomes and quality of life

   D) Mental health issues are less common in individuals with NCDs

9. Policy advocacy in health promotion aims to:

   A) Create barriers to healthy behaviors

   B) Promote policies that support a healthy environment

   C) Reduce public awareness about health issues

   D) Discourage collaboration between sectors

10. Technology and social media can be used in health promotion to:

A) Decrease communication with community members

B) Limit access to health information

C) Provide personalized feedback and support for healthy behaviors

D) Promote unhealthy lifestyle choices

Answers

1. C) Promoting a healthy diet

2. C) Provide immunity against specific infections

3. C) Promoting physical activity

4. B) Reporting unusual patterns of illness to health authorities

5. B) Reduced relevance of health initiatives

6. A) Regular screening and early intervention

7. B) Waterborne and foodborne diseases

8. C) It can improve treatment outcomes and quality of life

9. B) Promote policies that support a healthy environment

10. C) Provide personalized feedback and support for healthy behaviors

Chapter 3: Mental Health in the Community

3.1 Understanding Mental Health Issues

Mental health is an integral part of community health, influencing and being influenced by a variety of social, economic, and environmental factors. Understanding mental health issues involves recognizing the complexities of mental well-being, the spectrum of mental disorders, and the impact these conditions have on individuals and communities. This subchapter delves into the fundamentals of mental health issues, highlighting the importance of awareness, early identification, and the role of community support in addressing mental health challenges.

Mental health encompasses our emotional, psychological, and social well-being, affecting how we think, feel, and act. It also determines how we handle stress, relate to others, and make choices. Mental health issues can range from common disorders such as anxiety and depression to more severe conditions like schizophrenia and bipolar disorder. Recognizing the signs and symptoms of mental health issues is the first step toward addressing these challenges.

Prevalence and Impact

Mental health issues are common and can affect anyone, irrespective of age, gender, or social status. They can have a profound impact on the quality of life, affecting an individual's ability to work, engage in meaningful relationships, and participate in community life. The stigma and discrimination associated with mental illness further exacerbate the challenges faced by those affected, often hindering their access to care and support.

Causes of Mental Health Issues

The causes of mental health issues are multifaceted, involving a complex interplay of genetic, biological, environmental, and psychological factors. Life experiences, such as trauma or a history of abuse, can also contribute to the onset of mental health conditions. Social determinants, including poverty, unemployment, and social isolation, play a critical role in the prevalence and severity of mental health issues within communities.

The Role of Community Support

Communities play a crucial role in supporting individuals with mental health issues. Creating an environment that promotes mental well-being, reduces stigma, and encourages open discussions about mental health can facilitate early identification and intervention. Community-based support services, peer support groups, and mental health awareness campaigns are vital in fostering a supportive environment for those affected.

Early Identification and Intervention

Early identification and timely intervention are critical in managing mental health issues effectively. Community Health Workers (CHWs) and other community members can be trained to recognize the signs of mental distress and provide initial support or referral to mental health services. Schools, workplaces, and community centers can serve as important settings for mental health education and early detection initiatives.

Challenges in Addressing Mental Health Issues

Addressing mental health issues in the community faces several challenges, including limited resources, insufficient mental health professionals, and stigma. Overcoming these challenges requires a concerted effort from all stakeholders, including governments, healthcare providers, communities, and individuals, to invest in mental health services, education, and policies that promote mental well-being.

Understanding mental health issues is the foundation for building resilient communities that support mental well-being and provide the necessary resources and services to those in need. By promoting awareness, reducing stigma, and facilitating access to care, communities can make significant strides in improving the mental health of their members.

3.2 Strategies for Mental Health Support

Supporting mental health in the community requires a multifaceted approach that addresses both the needs of individuals with mental health conditions and the broader societal factors that influence mental well-being. Effective strategies for mental health support involve prevention, early intervention, treatment, and the integration of support services. This subchapter outlines key strategies that can be employed to support mental health in the community, emphasizing the role of collaborative efforts in enhancing mental health outcomes.

Promotion of Mental Well-being

The foundation of mental health support is the promotion of overall mental well-being. This includes raising awareness about mental health, educating the community on coping mechanisms and resilience-building strategies, and reducing stigma associated with mental health issues. Initiatives such as public awareness campaigns, school-based mental health education, and workplace wellness programs can contribute to a culture that values mental health.

Access to Mental Health Services

Improving access to mental health services is crucial in providing support to those in need. This involves not only increasing the availability of services but also making them accessible and affordable to all segments of the community. Integration of mental health services into primary healthcare settings, the provision of telehealth options, and the establishment of community mental health centers can enhance accessibility.

Community-Based Support Systems

Community-based support systems, including peer support groups, community health worker programs, and social services, play a vital role in supporting individuals with mental health issues. These services can offer practical assistance, emotional support, and linkage to other necessary services, fostering a network of care that supports recovery and resilience.

Crisis Intervention Services

For individuals experiencing a mental health crisis, immediate access to intervention services can be lifesaving. Crisis intervention services, such as hotlines, mobile crisis teams, and emergency mental health services, provide urgent support and can facilitate the transition to ongoing care.

Policy and Advocacy

Advocacy for policies that support mental health is essential in creating an enabling environment for mental health support. This includes policies that promote mental health education, protect the rights of individuals with mental health conditions, and ensure funding for mental health services. Advocacy efforts can also focus on addressing social determinants of mental health, such as housing, employment, and social inclusion.

Training and Education

Training and education for healthcare providers, community leaders, and the general public can enhance the community's capacity to support mental health. This includes training in mental health first aid, cultural competence, and the delivery of community-based mental health interventions.

Implementing these strategies requires collaboration among healthcare providers, community organizations, policymakers, and individuals. By working together, communities can build comprehensive support systems that address the varied aspects of mental health, from prevention and early intervention to treatment and recovery support.

3.3 Addressing Stigma and Discrimination

Stigma and discrimination against individuals with mental health issues are significant barriers to seeking help and receiving effective treatment. These negative attitudes and behaviors can come from society, within families, workplaces, and even among healthcare providers, further isolating individuals and exacerbating their conditions. Addressing stigma and discrimination is crucial for creating an inclusive community that supports mental health recovery and enables individuals to lead fulfilling lives. This subchapter explores strategies for combatting stigma and promoting a more understanding and supportive environment for those affected by mental health issues.

Education and Awareness

Raising awareness and educating the public about mental health is a fundamental step in changing perceptions and debunking myths surrounding mental health conditions. Initiatives that provide accurate information about the nature of mental health issues, their prevalence, and the reality of living with these conditions can help dispel fear and ignorance. Incorporating mental health education in schools, workplaces, and through media campaigns can reach wide audiences and foster a more informed and empathetic society.

Personal Stories and Advocacy

Sharing personal stories of those who have experienced mental health challenges can be a powerful tool in humanizing these conditions and reducing stigma. Advocacy by individuals with lived experience and their families can challenge stereotypes and highlight the possibility of recovery and a fulfilling life despite mental health issues. These narratives can inspire others to seek help and support mental health initiatives.

Community Involvement and Support Groups

Creating spaces for community support and involvement, such as support groups and community mental health initiatives, can promote a sense of belonging and acceptance for individuals with mental health issues. These platforms allow individuals to share experiences, offer and receive support, and work together to address stigma and discrimination in their communities.

Legislation and Policies

Implementing and enforcing laws that protect the rights of individuals with mental health conditions is crucial in addressing stigma and discrimination. Policies that ensure equal opportunities in employment, education, and access to healthcare services can help to eliminate systemic barriers and promote social inclusion. Advocacy for such policies is essential in creating a legal framework that supports equality and justice for individuals with mental health issues.

Training for Healthcare Providers and Professionals

Healthcare providers and professionals in various sectors (e.g., education, law enforcement) play a key role in shaping attitudes towards mental health. Training these individuals in mental health awareness, sensitivity, and the impact of stigma can improve their approach to individuals with mental health conditions, ensuring they provide support without prejudice or discrimination.

Promoting Mental Health as a Part of Overall Health

Integrating mental health into the broader conversation about health and wellness can help normalize mental health care and reduce stigma. Recognizing that mental health is as important as physical health encourages a more holistic approach to well-being and underscores the importance of addressing mental health issues with the same urgency and compassion as physical health problems.

Addressing stigma and discrimination is a continuous process that requires concerted efforts from all sectors of society. Through education, advocacy, supportive policies, and community engagement, it is possible to create a more inclusive and supportive environment for individuals facing mental health challenges.

3.4 Exercise: 10 MCQs with Answers at the End

This exercise aims to assess your understanding of the key concepts discussed in Chapter 3: Mental Health in the Community, focusing on understanding mental health issues, strategies for mental health support, and addressing stigma and discrimination. Reflect on the information presented in each section as you answer the questions. Correct answers provided at the end of the exercise will help gauge your grasp of these critical aspects of mental health support in community settings.

1. Mental health is crucial for:

   A) Physical health only

   B) Emotional, psychological, and social well-being

   C) Financial decision-making only

   D) Educational success only

2. A key strategy in supporting mental health in the community is:

A) Increasing social isolation

B) Reducing access to care

C) Promoting overall mental well-being

D) Encouraging self-diagnosis and treatment

3. Stigma and discrimination against individuals with mental health issues can lead to:

A) Improved self-esteem

B) Increased help-seeking behavior

C) Isolation and exacerbation of conditions

D) Greater social support

4. Effective crisis intervention services are characterized by:

A) Delayed response times

B) Immediate, urgent support

C) Lack of confidentiality

D) Focusing on long-term treatment only

5. Raising awareness and educating the public about mental health helps to:

A) Increase stigma and discrimination

B) Change perceptions and debunk myths

C) Discourage people from seeking help

D) Limit understanding of mental health issues

6. Community-based support systems for mental health might include:

A) Peer support groups and social services

B) Policies promoting social isolation

C) Decreased funding for mental health services

D) Encouraging individuals to cope on their own

7. Training healthcare providers in mental health sensitivity can:

A) Worsen their approach to care

B) Reduce prejudice and improve support

C) Increase discrimination in healthcare settings

D) Have no impact on care quality

8. Legislation that protects the rights of individuals with mental health conditions ensures:

   A) Reduced access to employment and education

   B) Increased public stigma

   C) Equal opportunities and social inclusion

   D) Less awareness about mental health issues

9. Sharing personal stories of mental health challenges helps to:

   A) Maintain stereotypes and fear

   B) Humanize conditions and reduce stigma

   C) Discourage others from seeking help

   D) Isolate individuals with mental health issues

10. A holistic approach to health includes:

   A) Ignoring mental health

   B) Viewing mental and physical health as separate

   C) Treating mental health with less urgency than physical health

   D) Recognizing mental health as important as physical health

Answers

1. B) Emotional, psychological, and social well-being

2. C) Promoting overall mental well-being

3. C) Isolation and exacerbation of conditions

4. B) Immediate, urgent support

5. B) Change perceptions and debunk myths

6. A) Peer support groups and social services

7. B) Reduce prejudice and improve support

8. C) Equal opportunities and social inclusion

9. B) Humanize conditions and reduce stigma

10. D) Recognizing mental health as important as physical health

Chapter 4: Nutrition and Public Health

4.1 The Importance of Nutrition in Health

Nutrition plays a pivotal role in public health, influencing individual well-being, community health outcomes, and overall societal productivity. The quality and quantity of food consumed not only affect physical growth and body functions but also have a profound impact on mental health, disease prevention, and life expectancy. This subchapter explores the fundamental importance of nutrition in health, shedding light on how dietary choices influence various aspects of human health and public health initiatives aimed at improving nutritional standards.

Nutritional Foundations for Health

Good nutrition is essential for maintaining healthy body functions, supporting growth and development, and providing energy for daily activities. It involves a balance of macronutrients (carbohydrates, proteins, and fats) and micronutrients (vitamins and minerals) to meet the body's needs. A well-balanced diet supports the immune system, aids in the prevention of non-communicable diseases such as diabetes and cardiovascular diseases, and contributes to overall health and well-being.

Impact on Disease Prevention

A direct link exists between nutrition and the prevention of chronic diseases. Diets high in saturated fats, trans fats, and added sugars can increase the risk of developing heart disease, obesity, and type 2 diabetes, while diets rich in fruits, vegetables, whole grains, and lean proteins can reduce this risk. Public health initiatives that promote healthy eating habits and increase access to nutritious foods are vital in combating the global burden of chronic diseases.

Nutrition and Mental Health

Emerging research highlights the significant impact of nutrition on mental health. Nutritional psychiatry studies how dietary patterns influence brain function, mood, and mental health disorders such as depression and anxiety. Adequate intake of essential nutrients, including omega-3 fatty acids, vitamins, and minerals, has been linked to improved mood and cognitive function, underscoring the importance of nutrition in mental health care.

Child Development and Nutrition

Nutrition is critically important during childhood and adolescence, as it affects growth, cognitive development, and future health outcomes. Malnutrition in early life can lead to long-term health issues, including stunted growth, poor academic performance, and increased susceptibility to diseases. Ensuring access to adequate nutrition for pregnant women, infants, and young children is a key focus of public health programs aimed at improving child health and development.

Public Health Strategies for Nutrition

Public health strategies to improve nutrition include creating policies that ensure food security, implementing nutrition education programs, and promoting healthy food environments. These strategies may involve regulating food labeling, restricting the marketing of unhealthy foods to children, and supporting local agriculture to increase the availability of fresh, nutritious foods. Community-based initiatives, such as school meal programs and community gardens, also play a crucial role in improving access to healthy foods and educating the public about the benefits of good nutrition.

The importance of nutrition in health cannot be overstated. By addressing nutritional needs and promoting healthy eating habits, public health initiatives can significantly improve health outcomes, reduce the prevalence of chronic diseases, and enhance the quality of life for individuals and communities. Recognizing and acting on the integral role of nutrition in health is essential for advancing public health goals and creating healthier societies.

4.2 Addressing Malnutrition

Malnutrition encompasses a wide range of nutritional imbalances, including undernutrition, micronutrient deficiencies, and overnutrition. It is a global health issue affecting millions of individuals, with profound implications for health, economic development, and societal well-being. Addressing malnutrition requires a comprehensive approach that targets its root causes and implements sustainable solutions. This subchapter delves into strategies for combating malnutrition in its various forms, emphasizing the critical role of public health interventions in mitigating its impact on communities worldwide.

Understanding the Scope of Malnutrition

Malnutrition is not merely a lack of sufficient food but a condition caused by a deficiency, excess, or imbalance in the intake of nutrients. Undernutrition, characterized by stunting, wasting, and underweight, remains a pressing issue in many low- and middle-income countries. Conversely, overnutrition, leading to overweight and obesity, is on the rise globally, contributing to a range of chronic diseases. Micronutrient deficiencies, often referred to as "hidden hunger," involve a lack of essential vitamins and minerals and can have severe health consequences, even in the absence of overt malnutrition symptoms.

Strategies for Prevention and Treatment

Effective strategies to combat malnutrition involve both preventive measures and targeted treatment interventions:

- **Nutrition Education and Awareness:** Education campaigns that provide information on balanced diets, nutritional requirements, and the importance of micronutrients can empower individuals to make healthier food choices. School-based nutrition programs can instill healthy eating habits from a young age.

- **Enhancing Food Security:** Ensuring access to a sufficient quantity of nutritious food is foundational in preventing malnutrition. Initiatives that support local food production, improve food distribution systems, and provide economic support to vulnerable populations are crucial.

- **Fortification and Supplementation:** Fortifying staple foods with essential vitamins and minerals can address micronutrient deficiencies on a large scale. Targeted supplementation programs, such as vitamin A supplementation for children and iron supplementation for pregnant women, are effective in reducing specific nutrient deficiencies.

- **Promoting Breastfeeding:** Exclusive breastfeeding for the first six months of life and continued breastfeeding alongside appropriate complementary foods up to two years of age or beyond provide critical nutrients and immune support to infants, protecting against childhood malnutrition.

- **Integrated Health Services:** Integrating nutrition services into broader health care systems can ensure that malnutrition prevention and treatment are part of routine health care. Screening for malnutrition and providing nutritional support should be standard components of maternal and child health services.

- **Community-Based Approaches:** Engaging communities in identifying and addressing malnutrition challenges can lead to more sustainable solutions. Community gardens, cooperative food programs, and peer-led education initiatives can enhance local food environments and promote nutritional well-being.

- **Policy and Advocacy:** Advocating for policies that address the root causes of malnutrition, including poverty, inequality, and lack of education, is essential. Policies that regulate the marketing of unhealthy foods, subsidize healthy food options, and support maternal and child health are examples of effective public health interventions.

Addressing malnutrition is a complex challenge that requires a coordinated effort among governments, non-governmental organizations, healthcare providers, and communities. By implementing a multifaceted approach that encompasses prevention, treatment, and policy advocacy, significant progress can be made in reducing the global burden of malnutrition and improving health outcomes for populations around the world.

4.3 Community-based Nutritional Interventions

Community-based nutritional interventions are essential strategies for improving public health outcomes by directly addressing the unique nutritional needs and challenges of specific populations. These interventions are designed to be accessible and culturally relevant, focusing on promoting healthy eating behaviors, preventing malnutrition, and addressing specific nutritional deficiencies within communities. This subchapter explores various types of community-based nutritional interventions and their impact on enhancing nutritional status and overall health.

Nutritional Education and Behavior Change Programs

These programs aim to increase knowledge about nutrition and encourage healthy eating habits through education and behavior change communication. Tailored to meet the cultural and socioeconomic context of the community, these interventions can include cooking classes, workshops on reading food labels, and campaigns promoting the consumption of fruits and vegetables. Engaging local leaders and community groups in these efforts ensures relevance and enhances the program's effectiveness.

School-based Nutrition Programs

Implementing nutrition programs in schools is a powerful way to reach children and adolescents with essential nutritional information and services. These can include school meals enriched with key nutrients, fruit and vegetable snack programs, and nutrition education integrated into the curriculum. Such initiatives not only improve nutritional status among students but also foster a culture of healthy eating from a young age.

Community Gardens and Urban Agriculture

Community gardens and urban agriculture projects provide fresh, nutritious produce to communities, particularly in urban areas where access to affordable healthy food can be limited.

These initiatives empower community members by involving them in the production of their food, promoting food security, and fostering social cohesion. They also serve as practical sites for nutrition education and can stimulate economic development within the community.

Maternal and Child Nutrition Programs

Programs focused on the nutritional needs of pregnant women, mothers, infants, and young children are critical for preventing malnutrition and its long-term consequences. These may include breastfeeding support groups, distribution of micronutrient supplements, and growth monitoring and promotion activities. Such interventions are vital for ensuring healthy growth and development and preventing stunting and wasting among children.

Food Assistance Programs

Food assistance programs, such as food banks, community pantries, and subsidized food schemes, play an important role in addressing food insecurity and its nutritional implications. By providing access to nutritious food items to those in need, these programs help mitigate the immediate impact of economic barriers on nutritional status.

Mobile Health and Nutrition Services

In areas with limited access to healthcare facilities, mobile health and nutrition services can bring vital nutritional support and information directly to communities. These services can include nutritional assessments, counseling, and the distribution of therapeutic foods or supplements to address specific deficiencies.

Public-Private Partnerships for Nutritional Improvement

Collaborations between governmental agencies, non-profit organizations, and the private sector can amplify the impact of community-based nutritional interventions. These partnerships can facilitate the fortification of staple foods, support the development of nutritious products targeted at low-income populations, and leverage technology to disseminate nutritional information widely.

Community-based nutritional interventions are key to addressing public health challenges related to nutrition. By focusing on the specific needs and contexts of communities, these interventions can effectively improve nutritional outcomes, reduce the prevalence of malnutrition, and contribute to the overall well-being and development of populations.

4.4 Exercise: 10 MCQs with Answers at the End

This exercise is designed to test your understanding of the concepts discussed in Chapter 4: Nutrition and Public Health, including the importance of nutrition, addressing malnutrition, and community-based nutritional interventions. Reflect on the information presented as you answer these questions. The correct answers provided at the end will help you assess your comprehension of nutritional strategies and their impact on public health.

1. Good nutrition is essential for:

   A) Energy for daily activities only

   B) Supporting growth and development

   C) Mental health only

   D) None of the above

2. Malnutrition includes:

   A) Undernutrition only

   B) Overnutrition only

   C) Micronutrient deficiencies only

   D) All of the above

3. School-based nutrition programs are important because they:

   A) Only provide free meals

   B) Improve nutritional status and foster healthy eating habits

   C) Are not effective in changing dietary behaviors

   D) Increase the burden on educational resources

4. Community gardens contribute to public health by:

   A) Decreasing access to fresh produce

   B) Providing a source of processed foods

   C) Enhancing food security and nutrition education

   D) Contributing to environmental pollution

5. Maternal and child nutrition programs focus on:

   A) Promoting adult health only

   B) The nutritional needs of teenagers

   C) Pregnant women, mothers, and young children

   D) Elderly populations only

6. Food assistance programs help mitigate:

   A) Economic prosperity

   B) Food insecurity and its nutritional implications

   C) The availability of fast food

   D) Nutritional education efforts

7. Mobile health and nutrition services are especially useful in:

   A) Urban areas with many healthcare facilities

   B) Areas with ample nutritional resources

   C) Communities with limited access to healthcare

D) High-income neighborhoods only

8. Fortification of staple foods is a strategy used in:

   A) Increasing the cost of food production

   B) Addressing specific micronutrient deficiencies

   C) Reducing the nutritional value of foods

   D) Promoting the consumption of junk food

9. Breastfeeding support groups are part of interventions aimed at:

   A) Discouraging breastfeeding

   B) Providing nutritional support for infants

   C) Reducing community cohesion

   D) Increasing infant exposure to diseases

10. Public-private partnerships in nutrition can:

   A) Only benefit the private sector

   B) Worsen the nutritional status of communities

   C) Amplify the impact of nutritional interventions

   D) Prevent any form of community-based nutrition program

Answers

1. B) Supporting growth and development

2. D) All of the above

3. B) Improve nutritional status and foster healthy eating habits

4. C) Enhancing food security and nutrition education

5. C) Pregnant women, mothers, and young children

6. B) Food insecurity and its nutritional implications

7. C) Communities with limited access to healthcare

8. B) Addressing specific micronutrient deficiencies

9. B) Providing nutritional support for infants

10. C) Amplify the impact of nutritional interventions

Chapter 5: Maternal and Child Health

5.1 Key Aspects of Maternal Health

Maternal health is a critical component of public health, focusing on the health of women during pregnancy, childbirth, and the postpartum period. Ensuring the health of mothers is crucial not only for their well-being but also for the health and survival of their children. This sub# Chapter explores the key aspects of maternal health, including the importance of prenatal care, management of maternal health conditions, the role of skilled birth attendance, and postpartum care, highlighting strategies to improve maternal health outcomes globally.

Prenatal Care

Prenatal care is vital for monitoring and promoting the health of the mother and developing fetus. Regular prenatal visits allow for the early detection and management of potential health issues, provide an opportunity for health education on nutrition, physical activity, and harmful substance avoidance, and prepare the mother for childbirth. Access to quality prenatal care is associated with reduced risks of maternal and infant mortality and morbidity.

Management of Maternal Health Conditions

Managing health conditions that can impact pregnancy outcomes, such as hypertension, diabetes, anemia, and infectious diseases, is a cornerstone of maternal health care. Effective management involves routine screening, timely intervention, and, where necessary, specialized care to prevent complications. Addressing these conditions requires a comprehensive health system approach that integrates maternal health services with broader health care services.

Skilled Birth Attendance

The presence of skilled health professionals during childbirth is essential for ensuring the health and safety of both the mother and the child. Skilled birth attendants are trained to manage normal deliveries and recognize the signs of complications that require emergency obstetric care. Increasing access to skilled birth attendance in all settings, especially in low-resource areas, is critical for reducing maternal and neonatal deaths.

Postpartum Care

The postpartum period, or the first six weeks after delivery, is a critical phase for monitoring the health of the mother and the newborn. Postpartum care services should include monitoring for complications, supporting breastfeeding and newborn care, managing mental health concerns such as postpartum depression, and providing family planning counseling. Adequate postpartum care is essential for the long-term health of both the mother and the child.

Challenges and Strategies for Improvement

Despite significant progress, maternal mortality and morbidity remain high in many parts of the world, particularly in low- and middle-income countries. Challenges include limited access to quality health services, lack of skilled health professionals, socio-economic and cultural barriers to care, and inadequate health infrastructure. Strategies for improvement focus on strengthening health systems, increasing investment in maternal and child health, enhancing community engagement and education, and implementing evidence-based interventions to address the specific needs of pregnant and postpartum women.

Improving maternal health is a multifaceted challenge that requires coordinated efforts across various sectors. By prioritizing maternal health in public health agendas and investing in comprehensive, culturally sensitive, and accessible care, significant strides can be made toward ensuring that all women have a healthy pregnancy and childbirth experience.

5.2 Child Health and Immunizations

Child health is a fundamental aspect of public health, focusing on the well-being of children from birth through adolescence. Immunizations play a critical role in child health, offering protection against serious and potentially fatal infectious diseases. This subchapter discusses the importance of child health and the role of immunizations in preventing disease, enhancing child survival rates, and contributing to the overall health of communities.

Importance of Child Health

Child health encompasses physical, mental, and social well-being. Ensuring the health of children involves not only addressing immediate health concerns but also establishing a foundation for healthy adulthood. Key areas in child health include nutrition, disease prevention, developmental monitoring, and the management of common childhood illnesses. Healthy children are more likely to become healthy adults, contributing to the economic and social strength of communities.

Immunizations: A Key Preventive Measure

Immunizations are among the most effective and cost-efficient public health interventions. Vaccines protect children from diseases such as measles, polio, tetanus, diphtheria, pertussis, and hepatitis B, among others. The World Health Organization (WHO) and various health agencies recommend vaccination schedules that cover essential vaccines for children and adolescents. By preventing infectious diseases, immunizations save millions of lives each year and prevent long-term disability associated with some infections.

Global and National Immunization Programs

Global initiatives, such as the Expanded Program on Immunization (EPI) by WHO, aim to ensure that all children worldwide receive essential vaccines. National immunization programs, supported by governments and international partners, strive to achieve high vaccination coverage to maintain herd immunity and prevent outbreaks of vaccine-preventable diseases. These programs often include campaigns to reach underserved and hard-to-reach populations.

Challenges to Immunization Efforts

Despite the success of immunization programs, challenges remain in reaching all children with life-saving vaccines. These challenges include logistical issues, such as vaccine storage and distribution; financial constraints; lack of awareness or misinformation about vaccines; and cultural or religious beliefs that lead to vaccine hesitancy. Addressing these challenges requires collaborative efforts among governments, healthcare providers, communities, and international organizations.

Strategies to Enhance Immunization Coverage

Improving immunization coverage involves several key strategies:

- Strengthening healthcare systems to ensure vaccines' availability, quality, and safe administration.

- Enhancing community engagement and education to increase awareness of the benefits of vaccination and address misconceptions.

- Investing in research and development to improve vaccine efficacy, develop new vaccines, and address emerging infectious diseases.

- Implementing innovative approaches to reach underserved populations, such as mobile vaccination clinics and the use of digital health technologies for tracking and reminders.

Child health and immunizations are intrinsically linked, with vaccines playing a pivotal role in preventing diseases that can impact children's health, development, and survival. By prioritizing immunization efforts and addressing the challenges to vaccine coverage, public health initiatives can continue to make significant strides in improving child health outcomes globally.

5.3 Preventing Mother-to-Child Transmission of Diseases

Preventing mother-to-child transmission (PMTCT) of diseases is a crucial public health strategy to protect the health of both mothers and their children. Certain infections can be transmitted from an infected mother to her baby during pregnancy, childbirth, or breastfeeding. Without intervention, diseases such as HIV, hepatitis B, syphilis, and others can significantly impact the health, development, and survival of infants. This subchapter explores the importance of preventing mother-to-child transmission, the key diseases of concern, and effective strategies for PMTCT.

Key Diseases of Concern

- **HIV:** Without treatment, the risk of mother-to-child transmission of HIV can be as high as 45%. PMTCT interventions can reduce this risk to below 5%.

- **Hepatitis B:** The virus can be transmitted from an infected mother to her infant at birth. Vaccination of newborns and the use of antiviral treatments during pregnancy can reduce the risk of transmission.

- **Syphilis:** Congenital syphilis can result from maternal syphilis infection during pregnancy, leading to stillbirth, neonatal death, or severe infections in newborns. Early screening and treatment during pregnancy can prevent transmission.

Strategies for PMTCT

- **Screening and Treatment During Pregnancy:** Early and routine screening for HIV, hepatitis B, syphilis, and other relevant infections during prenatal care allows for timely initiation of treatment to reduce the risk of transmission. For HIV, antiretroviral therapy (ART) significantly lowers the viral load in the mother, reducing the risk of transmission. For syphilis, antibiotic treatment is effective in preventing congenital syphilis.

- **Safe Birthing Practices:** Employing safe birthing practices and, when necessary, cesarean delivery can minimize the risk of transmission of certain infections during childbirth.

- **Immunization and Prophylaxis for Newborns:** Administering vaccines (e.g., hepatitis B vaccine) and prophylactic treatments (e.g., ART for newborns at risk of HIV) immediately after birth can further reduce the risk of mother-to-child transmission.

- **Breastfeeding Guidance:** For mothers with HIV, the decision to breastfeed involves weighing the risks of HIV transmission against the benefits of breastfeeding. In settings where safe alternatives to breastfeeding are not available, exclusive breastfeeding for the first six months, combined with maternal ART, is recommended to minimize the risk of transmission. For other infections, such as hepatitis B, breastfeeding is generally considered safe when the baby receives the hepatitis B vaccine and immunoglobulin if needed.

- **Community Education and Support:** Educating pregnant women and their families about the importance of PMTCT and supporting them throughout the process are critical for the success of these interventions. Community support can also help address stigma and barriers to accessing care.

The Role of Public Health Initiatives

Public health initiatives play a vital role in implementing and supporting PMTCT programs. This includes providing resources for screening and treatment, training healthcare providers, and ensuring access to necessary medications and vaccines. Collaborative efforts between governments, non-profit organizations, and international agencies are essential to expand access to PMTCT services and reduce the incidence of diseases transmitted from mother to child.

Preventing mother-to-child transmission of diseases is a key component of maternal and child health programs. Through effective screening, treatment, and support, it is possible to significantly reduce the risk of transmission and ensure healthier outcomes for mothers and their children.

5.5 Exercise: 10 MCQs with Answers at the End

This request seems to have been cut off or incomplete. If you were looking for a set of multiple-choice questions (MCQs) based on Chapter 5, covering maternal and child health, including key aspects of maternal health, child health and immunizations, and preventing mother-to-child transmission of diseases, I can certainly help with that. Here's a set of MCQs based on the discussed topics:

1. **Prenatal care is crucial for:**

   A) Monitoring maternal health only.

   B) Monitoring the fetus's development only.

   C) Monitoring both maternal health and the fetus's development.

   D) Providing vaccinations to the mother only.

2. **Effective management of maternal health conditions during pregnancy includes:**

   A) Routine screenings only.

   B) Timely interventions only.

C) Specialized care for complications only.

D) All of the above.

3. Skilled birth attendance is important because it:

A) Helps manage normal deliveries and recognize signs of complications.

B) Is required for all prenatal care.

C) Only provides psychological support to the mother.

D) Reduces the need for prenatal care.

4. Postpartum care is essential for:

A) The mother's health only.

B) The newborn's health only.

C) Both the mother's and newborn's health.

D) Addressing only nutritional needs.

5. Which of the following is a key preventive measure in child health?

A) Immunizations.

B) Limiting outdoor activities.

C) Restricting interaction with other children.

D) Avoiding routine check-ups.

6. **The Expanded Program on Immunization (EPI) aims to:**

   A) Provide vaccines to adults only.

   B) Ensure all children worldwide receive essential vaccines.

   C) Focus on treatment rather than prevention.

   D) Discourage the use of vaccines.

7. **Hepatitis B transmission from mother to child can be reduced through:**

   A) Avoiding breastfeeding.

   B) Immediate vaccination of the newborn.

   C) Antiviral treatments during adolescence.

   D) Limiting prenatal care.

8. **For HIV-positive mothers, which strategy is recommended to minimize the risk of mother-to-child transmission?**

   A) Avoiding treatment during pregnancy.

   B) Discontinuing ART after childbirth.

   C) Antiretroviral therapy (ART) during pregnancy and delivery.

   D) Exclusive breastfeeding without ART.

9. **Community education on PMTCT is important for:**

   A) Increasing stigma.

   B) Reducing the need for medical intervention.

C) Addressing barriers to accessing care.

D) Promoting exclusive formula feeding.

10. **Public health initiatives support PMTCT programs by:**

A) Providing resources for screening and treatment.

B) Training healthcare providers.

C) Ensuring access to necessary medications and vaccines.

D) All of the above.

Answers:

1. C) Monitoring both maternal health and the fetus's development.

2. D) All of the above.

3. A) Helps manage normal deliveries and recognize signs of complications.

4. C) Both the mother's and newborn's health.

5. A) Immunizations.

6. B) Ensure all children worldwide receive essential vaccines.

7. B) Immediate vaccination of the newborn.

8. C) Antiretroviral therapy (ART) during pregnancy and delivery.

9. C) Addressing barriers to accessing care.

10. D) All of the above.

Chapter 6: Managing Chronic Conditions

6.1 Overview of Chronic Diseases

Chronic diseases, also known as non-communicable diseases (NCDs), are long-term medical conditions that are generally progressive and are the leading cause of death and disability worldwide. They include a range of conditions such as cardiovascular diseases, diabetes, cancer, and chronic respiratory diseases. This subchapter provides an overview of chronic diseases, their impact on individual health and healthcare systems, and the importance of effective management strategies to mitigate their effects.

The Burden of Chronic Diseases

Chronic diseases are responsible for a significant portion of global morbidity and mortality, posing a major challenge to public health systems. Their prevalence is increasing, not only in high-income countries but also in low- and middle-income countries, largely due to changing lifestyles, aging populations, and increased exposure to risk factors such as tobacco use, unhealthy diets, physical inactivity, and excessive alcohol consumption.

Impact on Health Systems and Economies

The management of chronic diseases requires ongoing medical care and can lead to significant healthcare costs for both individuals and health systems. These diseases often necessitate long-term treatment and care, including medications, therapies, and possible hospitalizations, contributing to the economic burden on healthcare systems. Additionally, chronic conditions can impact an individual's ability to work, further affecting economic productivity and quality of life.

Risk Factors

Understanding the risk factors for chronic diseases is crucial for prevention and management. While some factors, such as age and genetics, are non-modifiable, many others are related to lifestyle choices and environmental exposures. Modifiable risk factors include:

- Tobacco use

- Unhealthy diets

- Physical inactivity

- Harmful use of alcohol

- Exposure to air pollution

Prevention and Management

Preventing chronic diseases and managing existing conditions require a comprehensive approach that includes:

- **Public Health Interventions:** These aim to reduce exposure to risk factors through policies and programs that promote healthy lifestyles and environments.

- **Individual Lifestyle Changes:** Encouraging individuals to adopt healthier behaviors, such as eating a balanced diet, engaging in regular physical activity, avoiding tobacco and excessive alcohol consumption, and managing stress.

- **Early Detection and Screening:** Regular screening for risk factors and early stages of disease can facilitate early intervention and prevent progression.

- **Integrated Care:** Effective management of chronic conditions often involves coordinated care among various healthcare providers and services, focusing on patient-centered approaches that address the full spectrum of the patient's needs.

The Role of Technology and Innovation

Advancements in technology and healthcare innovation play a significant role in managing chronic diseases. Telemedicine, digital health tools, and personalized medicine are increasingly being used to improve access to care, monitor health indicators, and tailor treatments to individual patient needs.

Chronic diseases represent a complex challenge that requires a multifaceted response from healthcare systems, governments, communities, and individuals. Through targeted public health initiatives, lifestyle interventions, early detection, and integrated care models, it is possible to reduce the impact of chronic diseases on individuals and societies, improving health outcomes and quality of life.

6.2 Community Management of Diabetes

Diabetes, a chronic metabolic disorder characterized by high blood sugar levels, is a major public health issue affecting millions worldwide. Its management is crucial not only for the well-being of individuals but also for the sustainability of healthcare systems. Community management of diabetes involves a comprehensive approach that includes prevention, early detection, education, and support for individuals with diabetes. This subchapter focuses on strategies for effective community management of diabetes, aiming to reduce its incidence and mitigate complications.

Prevention and Early Detection

Preventing diabetes and identifying it early in individuals at risk are key components of community management. Prevention strategies involve:

- **Promoting Healthy Lifestyles:** Encouraging regular physical activity, healthy eating, and maintaining a healthy weight can significantly reduce the risk of type 2 diabetes.

- **Screening and Risk Assessment:** Regular screening for prediabetes and risk assessments in primary care settings can identify individuals at high risk, allowing for early intervention.

Education and Self-Management

Education is a cornerstone of diabetes management, empowering individuals to take control of their condition. Effective community programs include:

- **Diabetes Education Programs:** Providing individuals with knowledge about diabetes management, including monitoring blood sugar levels, understanding medication, and recognizing signs of complications.

- **Self-Management Support:** Offering tools and resources for self-monitoring, dietary planning, and physical activity guidance helps individuals manage their diabetes more effectively.

Access to Care and Treatment

Ensuring access to medical care and treatment is essential for effective diabetes management. Community strategies include:

- **Integration of Services:** Integrating diabetes care into primary healthcare services ensures individuals have regular access to care.

- **Subsidized Medications and Supplies:** Providing affordable medications and diabetes management supplies, such as glucose meters and test strips, supports ongoing management.

Community Support Systems

Building supportive environments and networks within communities aids in the management of diabetes by:

- **Support Groups:** Facilitating peer support groups where individuals with diabetes can share experiences and coping strategies.

- **Community Health Workers:** Utilizing community health workers to provide education, support, and referrals enhances access to care and resources.

Addressing Social Determinants

Recognizing and addressing the social determinants of health that contribute to diabetes risk, such as poverty, education, and access to healthy foods, are important aspects of community management. Strategies include:

- **Food Access Programs:** Initiatives like community gardens, farmers' markets with subsidized options, and nutrition assistance programs improve access to healthy foods.

- **Healthy Environment Initiatives:** Creating safe and accessible places for physical activity, such as parks and walking trails, promotes regular exercise.

Monitoring and Evaluation

Ongoing monitoring and evaluation of community management programs ensure their effectiveness and allow for adjustments based on community needs. Collecting data on diabetes prevalence, management outcomes, and program participation provides valuable insights for continuous improvement.

Community management of diabetes requires a multi-sectoral approach that combines medical care with preventive measures, education, support, and policies to address broader determinants of health. By engaging healthcare providers, community organizations, individuals with diabetes, and the wider community, it is possible to create comprehensive strategies that improve diabetes outcomes and enhance the quality of life for those affected.

6.3 Hypertension: Prevention and Management

Hypertension, or high blood pressure, is a common chronic condition that significantly increases the risk of heart disease, stroke, and other serious health issues. Its management and prevention are crucial for reducing the burden of cardiovascular diseases and improving population health. Effective prevention and management of hypertension require a multifaceted approach that encompasses lifestyle interventions, community engagement, access to healthcare, and patient education. This subchapter outlines strategies to combat hypertension within communities, aiming to lower prevalence rates and enhance overall health outcomes.

Prevention Strategies

- **Healthy Lifestyle Promotion:** Encouraging a healthy lifestyle is foundational in preventing hypertension. This includes maintaining a balanced diet rich in fruits, vegetables, whole grains, and low in saturated fats and sodium; engaging in regular physical activity; limiting alcohol consumption; and avoiding tobacco use. Community programs can support these behaviors through educational campaigns, fitness programs, and nutrition workshops.

- **Screening and Risk Assessment:** Regular blood pressure screenings and risk assessments can identify individuals at risk of developing hypertension early. Community health fairs, primary care settings, and workplaces can serve as effective venues for these screenings, facilitating early intervention.

Management Approaches

- **Access to Healthcare Services:** Ensuring that individuals with hypertension have access to regular healthcare services is critical for effective management. This includes routine monitoring of blood pressure, medication management, and access to healthcare professionals for advice and support.

- **Patient Education:** Educating patients about hypertension, including how to monitor their blood pressure at home, the importance of medication adherence, and recognizing signs of complications, empowers individuals to take an active role in managing their condition.

- **Community Support Systems:** Support groups and community health initiatives can provide additional resources and support for individuals with hypertension. Peer support can be particularly effective in encouraging lifestyle changes and medication adherence.

- **Addressing Social Determinants:** Social determinants of health, such as socioeconomic status, education, and access to healthy foods, can influence hypertension risk and management. Community interventions that address these determinants, such as food access programs and health education, can improve hypertension outcomes.

- **Policy Interventions:** Public health policies that create environments supportive of healthy choices can contribute to hypertension prevention. Examples include regulations to reduce sodium in processed foods, taxes on sugary beverages, and the development of safe, accessible areas for physical activity.

Technology and Innovation in Hypertension Management

- **Digital Health Tools:** The use of digital health tools, such as smartphone apps for tracking blood pressure and lifestyle changes, telehealth services for remote consultations, and wearable devices for continuous monitoring, can enhance hypertension management by providing patients and healthcare providers with real-time data and facilitating personalized care.

- **Community Engagement:** Engaging the community in hypertension awareness and prevention efforts can amplify the impact of these strategies. This includes partnerships with local organizations, schools, and businesses to promote health education and support healthy environments.

Effective prevention and management of hypertension require collaborative efforts from healthcare providers, patients, community organizations, and policymakers. By implementing comprehensive strategies that address lifestyle factors, healthcare access, education, and social determinants of health, communities can significantly reduce the prevalence of hypertension and its associated health risks.

6.4 Exercise: 10 MCQs with Answers at the End

Creating a set of MCQs focusing on the comprehensive understanding of managing chronic conditions, specifically targeting diabetes and hypertension, encapsulates the essence of preventive strategies, management, and community engagement. Here's a tailored set of questions along with the answers:

1. **What is a primary goal in the community management of diabetes?**

   A) To increase sugar consumption in diets

   B) To reduce the incidence and mitigate complications

   C) To discourage physical activity

   D) None of the above

2. **Which lifestyle change is NOT recommended for diabetes prevention?**

A) Increasing physical activity

B) Consuming a balanced diet rich in fruits and vegetables

C) Maintaining a sedentary lifestyle

D) Avoiding excessive sugar intake

3. **Regular screening for diabetes is important because it:**

A) Can identify the disease in its early stages when it is most treatable

B) Is only necessary for individuals over 65

C) Should be done only when symptoms appear

D) None of the above

4. **Community health workers contribute to diabetes management by:**

A) Only providing medical treatment

B) Offering education, support, and referrals

C) Discouraging individuals from seeking healthcare

D) Ignoring the social determinants of health

5. **A key strategy in hypertension prevention is:**

A) Reducing salt intake

B) Increasing alcohol consumption

C) Avoiding all physical activities

D) None of the above

6. **Which of the following is a benefit of integrating hypertension management into primary healthcare?**

A) Decreases access to care

B) Ensures individuals receive consistent and comprehensive care

C) Limits the availability of blood pressure monitoring

D) Increases the cost of treatment

7. **Effective hypertension management often includes:**

A) Ignoring blood pressure readings

B) Regular physical activity and dietary changes

C) Increasing salt and fat intake in the diet

D) All of the above

8. **One way to address the social determinants of health in managing hypertension is:**

A) Limiting access to healthcare based on socioeconomic status

B) Improving access to healthy foods and safe places for exercise

C) Encouraging a sedentary lifestyle

D) None of the above

9. **Why are support groups beneficial for individuals with chronic conditions like diabetes and hypertension?**

A) They provide a platform for sharing misinformation

B) They discourage adherence to treatment plans

C) They offer emotional support and practical advice for management

D) They are not beneficial

10. **Monitoring and evaluation of community management programs are important because they:**

A) Ensure the programs are ineffective

B) Provide insights for continuous improvement

C) Are not necessary for chronic disease management

D) Increase the risk of complications

Answers:

1. B) To reduce the incidence and mitigate complications

2. C) Maintaining a sedentary lifestyle

3. A) Can identify the disease in its early stages when it is most treatable

4. B) Offering education, support, and referrals

5. A) Reducing salt intake

6. B) Ensures individuals receive consistent and comprehensive care

7. B) Regular physical activity and dietary changes

8. B) Improving access to healthy foods and safe places for exercise

9. C) They offer emotional support and practical advice for management

10. B) Provide insights for continuous improvement

Chapter 7: Infectious Disease Control

7.1 Strategies for Controlling Infectious Diseases

Infectious diseases remain a major public health challenge worldwide, causing significant morbidity and mortality. The control of infectious diseases involves a multifaceted approach that includes surveillance, prevention, early detection, and effective response to outbreaks. This subchapter outlines the essential strategies employed in the control of infectious diseases, emphasizing their importance in protecting public health and preventing the spread of infections.

Surveillance and Reporting Systems

Effective infectious disease control begins with robust surveillance and reporting systems. These systems track the incidence and spread of diseases, providing critical data for early warning and response. Public health authorities rely on this information to identify outbreaks, monitor disease trends, and allocate resources efficiently.

Vaccination Programs

Vaccination is one of the most effective tools for preventing infectious diseases. Immunization programs aim to achieve and maintain high coverage rates within populations, providing herd immunity and preventing outbreaks of vaccine-preventable diseases such as measles, polio, and influenza.

Public Health Education and Awareness

Educating the public about infectious diseases and how to prevent them is crucial. Health education campaigns can promote behaviors that reduce the risk of infection, such as hand hygiene, safe food handling, and the use of protective measures during outbreaks.

Infection Prevention and Control (IPC) Measures

IPC measures in healthcare settings and the community are essential for preventing the transmission of infectious diseases. These measures include the use of personal protective equipment (PPE), hand hygiene practices, environmental cleaning, and the isolation of infected individuals.

Antimicrobial Stewardship

The rational use of antimicrobials, including antibiotics, is critical in controlling infectious diseases and combating antibiotic resistance. Antimicrobial stewardship programs aim to optimize the use of antimicrobials to treat infections while minimizing the risk of resistance development.

Vector Control

For diseases transmitted by vectors such as mosquitoes, ticks, and fleas, vector control strategies are vital. These strategies include the use of insecticide-treated bed nets, environmental management to eliminate breeding sites, and the application of insecticides.

International Cooperation and Coordination

Infectious diseases do not respect borders, making international cooperation essential for effective control. Collaborative efforts include sharing surveillance data, coordinating response efforts to outbreaks, and supporting global health initiatives aimed at infectious disease control.

Research and Development

Investment in research and development is crucial for advancing the understanding of infectious diseases, developing new vaccines and treatments, and improving diagnostic tools. Ongoing research is essential for responding to emerging infectious diseases and adapting control strategies to changing epidemiological patterns.

Community Engagement

Engaging communities in infectious disease control efforts ensures the success of interventions. Community participation can enhance surveillance, increase vaccination uptake, and promote adherence to IPC measures and other preventive behaviors.

Effective control of infectious diseases requires a comprehensive approach that integrates various strategies across different levels of the healthcare system and the community. By implementing these strategies, public health authorities can protect populations from the impact of infectious diseases, reduce the burden on healthcare systems, and contribute to global health security.

7.2 HIV/AIDS: Community-Based Approaches

The HIV/AIDS epidemic remains a significant public health challenge, particularly in regions with high prevalence rates. Community-based approaches to HIV/AIDS prevention, treatment, and care have proven effective in reaching populations most at risk and providing services in a more accessible, acceptable, and sustainable manner. This subchapter explores various community-based approaches to managing the HIV/AIDS epidemic, emphasizing their importance in reducing transmission rates, improving treatment outcomes, and supporting affected individuals and communities.

Prevention and Education

Community-based prevention and education initiatives are crucial in raising awareness about HIV transmission modes, promoting safer sexual behaviors, and encouraging regular testing. These initiatives often involve:

- Peer education programs that leverage the influence of community members to disseminate information.

- Distribution of condoms and promotion of safe sex practices.

- Educational campaigns targeting specific at-risk populations, including young people, sex workers, and intravenous drug users.

Voluntary Testing and Counseling

Offering voluntary HIV testing and counseling in community settings increases the likelihood of individuals learning their HIV status and receiving necessary support. Mobile testing units, home-based testing services, and community health centers can provide confidential and convenient testing options, coupled with pre- and post-test counseling.

Antiretroviral Treatment (ART) Access

Expanding access to ART through community-based distribution points and support systems enhances treatment adherence and outcomes. Community health workers can play a pivotal role in delivering medications, monitoring adherence, and providing education on managing side effects.

Support Groups and Networks

Community support groups and networks offer critical psychosocial support to people living with HIV/AIDS. These groups provide a platform for sharing experiences, coping strategies, and mutual encouragement. They can also advocate for the rights of people living with HIV/AIDS, reducing stigma and discrimination within the community.

Care and Support Services

Community-based care and support services address the holistic needs of people living with HIV/AIDS, including medical, nutritional, and emotional support. Home-based care programs, nutritional support, and palliative care services can improve the quality of life for those affected by HIV/AIDS.

Harm Reduction Programs

For populations at high risk of HIV transmission through intravenous drug use, harm reduction programs provide essential services, such as needle exchange programs and access to opioid substitution therapy, to reduce the risk of HIV transmission.

Partnerships and Collaboration

Effective community-based HIV/AIDS approaches rely on partnerships between governments, non-governmental organizations (NGOs), healthcare providers, and the communities themselves. Collaborative efforts ensure that interventions are well-coordinated, culturally appropriate, and sustainable.

Addressing Social Determinants

Community-based initiatives also address the social determinants of health that contribute to the risk of HIV infection, such as poverty, gender inequality, and lack of education. Efforts to improve economic opportunities, empower women, and enhance educational access are integral to reducing vulnerability to HIV/AIDS.

Community-based approaches to HIV/AIDS are essential for reaching marginalized and hard-to-reach populations, providing holistic care and support, and building resilience within communities. By engaging community members in prevention, treatment, and care efforts, these approaches contribute significantly to controlling the HIV/AIDS epidemic and improving the lives of those affected.

7.3 Tuberculosis and Malaria in Community Health

Tuberculosis (TB) and malaria are two infectious diseases that significantly impact global health, especially in low- and middle-income countries. Community health strategies play a crucial role in the prevention, detection, and management of these diseases, contributing to their control and eventual elimination. This subchapter explores the challenges and community-based approaches to managing tuberculosis and malaria, highlighting their importance in enhancing public health outcomes.

Tuberculosis (TB)

TB is a bacterial infection that primarily affects the lungs but can also impact other parts of the body. Despite being preventable and curable, TB remains one of the top infectious disease killers globally. Community health strategies for TB control include:

- **Awareness and Education:** Raising awareness about TB signs and symptoms, transmission modes, and the importance of completing treatment regimens. Education campaigns can empower communities to seek early diagnosis and adhere to treatment.

- **Active Case Finding:** Community health workers conducting door-to-door visits or setting up local screening camps to identify TB cases early, especially in high-risk populations.

- **Directly Observed Therapy (DOT):** Implementing DOT strategies where health workers or trained community volunteers observe patients taking their TB medication, ensuring adherence to the treatment course.

- **Nutritional Support:** Providing nutritional support to TB patients, as malnutrition can exacerbate the disease and hinder recovery.

- **Integration with HIV Services:** Given the high co-infection rate of TB and HIV, integrating TB screening and treatment with HIV services ensures comprehensive care for affected individuals.

Malaria

Malaria, caused by Plasmodium parasites transmitted through the bite of infected Anopheles mosquitoes, continues to cause significant morbidity and mortality in tropical and subtropical regions. Community-based malaria control efforts include:

- **Vector Control:** Implementing community-wide vector control measures, such as the use of insecticide-treated bed nets (ITNs) and indoor residual spraying (IRS), to reduce mosquito populations and interrupt transmission.

- **Environmental Management:** Engaging communities in environmental management practices to eliminate mosquito breeding sites, such as standing water.

- **Education on Prevention:** Educating communities on malaria prevention practices and the correct use of ITNs and other protective measures.

- **Prompt Diagnosis and Treatment:** Promoting access to rapid diagnostic tests (RDTs) and effective antimalarial medications in community settings to ensure timely treatment of malaria cases.

- **Community Participation:** Mobilizing community participation in malaria control activities, such as bed net distribution campaigns and awareness programs, to foster a sense of ownership and responsibility.

Challenges and Solutions

Both TB and malaria present unique challenges, including drug resistance, access to diagnostic and treatment services, and maintaining sustained funding for control efforts. Solutions involve strengthening health systems, investing in research and development for new diagnostics, drugs, and vaccines, and fostering global and local partnerships to support community-based initiatives.

Community engagement and tailored strategies that consider the local context, resources, and needs are essential for the effective management of TB and malaria. By empowering communities to take an active role in prevention, detection, and treatment, significant progress can be made toward controlling these diseases and improving overall public health.

7.4 Exercise: 10 MCQs with Answers at the End

Creating a set of multiple-choice questions (MCQs) based on the comprehensive understanding of infectious disease control, specifically focusing on strategies for controlling infectious diseases, community-based approaches to HIV/AIDS, and tackling tuberculosis and malaria in community health, offers a valuable tool for assessing knowledge and reinforcing learning. Here's a tailored set of questions along with the answers:

1. Effective infectious disease control begins with:

A) Vaccine development only.

B) Robust surveillance and reporting systems.

C) Treating infected individuals only.

D) Ignoring asymptomatic cases.

2. Which strategy is NOT part of the community-based approach to HIV/AIDS?

A) Distributing antiretroviral therapy at community centers.

B) Encouraging the sharing of needles to reduce costs.

C) Offering voluntary HIV testing and counseling.

D) Promoting safe sex practices through education.

3. For tuberculosis (TB) control, Directly Observed Therapy (DOT) is important because it:

A) Reduces the need for patient education.

B) Ensures patients complete their treatment regimen.

C) Allows patients to self-administer medication without supervision.

D) Is only used in hospital settings.

4. In malaria control, the use of insecticide-treated bed nets (ITNs) aims to:

A) Increase mosquito populations.

B) Reduce human-mosquito contact during peak biting hours.

C) Diagnose malaria infections.

D) Treat malaria symptoms.

5. A critical challenge in the management of TB and malaria is:

A) The effectiveness of traditional medicines.

B) Access to clean water.

C) Drug resistance.

D) Overuse of insect repellents.

6. Community engagement in infectious disease control:

A) Decreases public awareness.

B) Is unnecessary for disease prevention.

C) Fosters a sense of ownership and responsibility.

D) Increases the spread of infections.

7. Antimicrobial stewardship programs aim to:

A) Promote the overuse of antibiotics.

B) Optimize the use of antimicrobials to combat resistance.

C) Discourage the development of new antibiotics.

D) Limit the treatment options for viral infections.

8. An effective way to address HIV/AIDS stigma in communities is through:

A) Avoiding discussions about HIV/AIDS.

B) Sharing personal stories of those living with HIV/AIDS.

C) Segregating individuals with HIV/AIDS.

D) Decreasing funding for HIV/AIDS education.

9. Which is a key component of early detection in infectious disease control?

A) Ignoring mild symptoms.

B) Regular screening and risk assessments.

C) Waiting for an outbreak to begin testing.

D) Focusing on treatment only, not prevention.

10. **Vector control measures, such as environmental management, are essential in controlling:**

A) Non-communicable diseases.

B) Mental health disorders.

C) Malaria.

D) Diabetes.

Answers:

1. B) Robust surveillance and reporting systems.

2. B) Encouraging the sharing of needles to reduce costs.

3. B) Ensures patients complete their treatment regimen.

4. B) Reduce human-mosquito contact during peak biting hours.

5. C) Drug resistance.

6. C) Fosters a sense of ownership and responsibility.

7. B) Optimize the use of antimicrobials to combat resistance.

8. B) Sharing personal stories of those living with HIV/AIDS.

9. B) Regular screening and risk assessments.

10. C) Malaria.

Chapter 8: Environmental Health and Safety

8.1 Water, Sanitation, and Hygiene (WASH)

Water, Sanitation, and Hygiene (WASH) are foundational pillars of public health, directly impacting the prevention of diseases and the promotion of health and well-being in communities worldwide. Access to clean water, proper sanitation, and good hygiene practices are essential for maintaining health, preventing waterborne and infectious diseases, and contributing to socioeconomic development. This subchapter delves into the importance of WASH, its impact on public health, and strategies to improve WASH services and practices.

Importance of WASH

- **Disease Prevention:** Many diseases, including diarrhea, cholera, dysentery, and typhoid, are waterborne and can be significantly reduced through improved WASH practices. Proper sanitation and hygiene interrupt the transmission of these diseases.

- **Nutritional Impact:** WASH has a direct impact on nutrition. Contaminated water and poor sanitation contribute to malnutrition and stunting in children by causing frequent episodes of diarrhea and other infections.

- **Economic Benefits:** Investing in WASH initiatives leads to economic gains by reducing healthcare costs associated with treating waterborne diseases and improving productivity through better health.

- **Women and Children's Health:** WASH programs have profound implications for the health and safety of women and children, who are often most vulnerable to WASH-related diseases. Access to safe toilets and water sources also contributes to the dignity, privacy, and safety of women and girls.

Strategies for Improving WASH Services

- **Infrastructure Development:** Building and maintaining infrastructure for safe water supply and sanitation facilities, including toilets and sewage systems, are crucial for improving WASH outcomes.

- **Behavioral Change Campaigns:** Education and awareness campaigns that promote hygiene practices, such as handwashing with soap, safe food handling, and the proper use of sanitation facilities, are essential for sustaining health benefits.

- **Community-Led Total Sanitation (CLTS):** CLTS approaches focus on mobilizing communities to completely eliminate open defecation through community participation and the construction of latrines without external financial subsidies.

- **Policy and Governance:** Effective policies and strong governance are needed to allocate resources, regulate WASH services, and ensure equitable access for all segments of the population, including the most vulnerable.

- **Innovation and Technology:** Utilizing innovative technologies and approaches, such as solar-powered water purification systems and eco-friendly sanitation solutions, can enhance the sustainability and efficiency of WASH services.

- **Partnerships:** Collaborations between governments, NGOs, community organizations, and the private sector can leverage resources, expertise, and advocacy efforts to expand and improve WASH services.

Challenges to WASH Implementation

Despite progress, significant challenges remain in providing universal access to WASH services. These include funding gaps, climate change impacts on water availability, conflicts and displacement disrupting access to WASH facilities, and the need for behavior change to adopt and maintain hygiene practices.

Addressing these challenges requires a concerted and collaborative effort from all stakeholders involved in public health, environmental protection, and development. By prioritizing WASH as a key public health issue, communities can make significant strides in improving health outcomes, protecting the environment, and achieving sustainable development goals.

8.2 Managing Environmental Risks to Health

Environmental risks, including pollution, chemical exposures, and climate change, significantly impact public health. Effective management of these risks requires a multidisciplinary approach that combines policy, community action, and individual behavior changes. This subchapter delves into strategies for managing environmental risks to health, emphasizing the importance of safeguarding communities and ecosystems.

Identifying and Assessing Environmental Risks

The first step in managing environmental risks involves identifying and assessing the sources of risk, such as air and water pollution, toxic waste, and hazardous chemicals. Risk assessments help determine the potential impact on public health and guide the development of targeted interventions.

Regulation and Policy Enforcement

Implementing and enforcing environmental regulations is critical for reducing exposure to harmful substances and practices. Policies that limit emissions from industrial and vehicular sources, regulate the use and disposal of hazardous materials, and promote sustainable land use can mitigate environmental health risks.

Monitoring and Surveillance

Ongoing monitoring of environmental conditions and health outcomes is essential for tracking progress and identifying emerging risks. Surveillance systems can alert public health officials to outbreaks of diseases related to environmental factors, enabling timely responses.

Community Engagement and Education

Educating communities about environmental health risks and engaging them in risk reduction activities empowers individuals to take action. Community-led initiatives, such as clean-up campaigns, tree planting, and recycling programs, can significantly improve local environmental conditions.

Climate Change Adaptation and Mitigation

Climate change poses a broad range of health risks, including those related to extreme weather events, vector-borne diseases, and food security. Adaptation strategies, such as developing resilient infrastructure and emergency preparedness plans, are necessary to protect public health. Mitigation efforts, including reducing greenhouse gas emissions and increasing carbon sequestration, are crucial for long-term health and safety.

Promoting Sustainable Practices

Encouraging sustainable environmental and economic practices among industries, agriculture, and communities reduces environmental health risks. Sustainable practices include reducing waste, conserving water, using clean energy sources, and adopting eco-friendly farming techniques.

Integrating Environmental Health into Public Health Planning

Incorporating environmental health considerations into broader public health planning and healthcare provision ensures a comprehensive approach to health and wellbeing. This integration can enhance the effectiveness of interventions aimed at reducing environmental risks.

Advancing Environmental Health Research

Investment in research is vital for understanding the complex relationships between environmental exposures and health outcomes. Research can inform the development of new technologies and interventions to mitigate environmental risks.

Managing environmental risks to health requires a concerted effort from governments, non-governmental organizations, businesses, communities, and individuals. By implementing comprehensive strategies that address the root causes of environmental health risks and promote sustainable practices, it is possible to protect public health and ensure a healthier future for all.

8.3 Disaster Preparedness and Response

Disasters, whether natural or man-made, pose significant threats to public health, safety, and well-being. Effective disaster preparedness and response mechanisms are crucial for minimizing the impact of disasters on communities and ensuring a swift recovery. This subchapter focuses on the key components of disaster preparedness and response, highlighting the role of various stakeholders in building resilience and enhancing the capacity to cope with disasters.

Disaster Preparedness

Preparedness involves planning and preparing for disasters before they occur to reduce their impact. Key elements include:

- **Risk Assessment:** Identifying potential hazards and assessing risks to prioritize preparedness efforts.

- **Emergency Planning:** Developing comprehensive emergency plans that detail roles, responsibilities, and actions before, during, and after a disaster.

- **Public Education and Training:** Educating the public about disaster risks and preparedness actions, and training emergency response teams and volunteers.

- **Infrastructure Resilience:** Strengthening infrastructure to withstand disasters, including buildings, transportation systems, and utility networks.

- **Resource Allocation:** Ensuring the availability of necessary resources, such as emergency supplies, equipment, and funding.

- **Early Warning Systems:** Implementing systems to detect and provide timely warnings about impending disasters to mitigate their impact.

Disaster Response

Response actions are taken during and immediately after a disaster to save lives, reduce health impacts, and support affected communities. Key aspects include:

- **Rapid Assessment:** Quickly assessing the extent of the disaster and the immediate needs of affected populations.

- **Search and Rescue:** Mobilizing teams to locate and rescue individuals trapped or injured by the disaster.

- **Medical Assistance:** Providing emergency medical care and support, including trauma care, mental health services, and disease prevention efforts.

- **Shelter and Relief:** Establishing temporary shelters and distributing relief supplies, such as food, water, and clothing.

- **Communication:** Maintaining clear and effective communication with the public and among response teams to coordinate efforts and disseminate important information.

Recovery and Rehabilitation

Recovery involves restoring communities to their pre-disaster state or better, focusing on long-term rebuilding and rehabilitation. This includes:

- **Reconstruction of Infrastructure:** Rebuilding damaged infrastructure with improvements to reduce future disaster risks.

- **Economic and Social Recovery:** Supporting the economic recovery of affected areas and addressing social impacts, including displacement and mental health issues.

- **Environmental Restoration:** Addressing environmental damage caused by the disaster and implementing measures to prevent future environmental risks.

- **Lessons Learned and Policy Development:** Evaluating the response to identify lessons learned and inform the development of policies and practices for better future disaster preparedness and response.

Effective disaster preparedness and response require a coordinated effort among governments, non-governmental organizations, communities, and international partners. By fostering a culture of preparedness, investing in resilient infrastructure, and ensuring rapid and efficient response mechanisms, societies can reduce the devastating impact of disasters and enhance community resilience.

8.4 Exercise: 10 MCQs with Answers at the End

Creating a set of multiple-choice questions (MCQs) based on Chapter 8, focusing on Environmental Health and Safety, including Water, Sanitation, and Hygiene (WASH), managing environmental risks to health, and disaster preparedness and response, offers a concise method to test comprehension and reinforce key concepts. Here's a set of MCQs with the answers provided:

1. Effective WASH programs are essential for preventing:

A) Non-communicable diseases.

B) Physical injuries.

C) Infectious diseases.

D) Mental health disorders.

2. A key strategy in managing environmental risks to health is:

A) Increasing industrial emissions.

B) Regulation and policy enforcement.

C) Reducing public green spaces.

D) Promoting the use of single-use plastics.

3. In disaster preparedness, risk assessment is important for:

A) Identifying potential hazards and assessing risks.

B) Decreasing community engagement.

C) Ignoring infrastructure resilience.

D) Focusing solely on economic recovery.

4. Which is NOT a component of disaster response?

A) Rapid assessment.

B) Search and rescue operations.

C) Immediate reconstruction of infrastructure.

D) Medical assistance.

5. Public education and training in disaster preparedness aim to:

A) Reduce the effectiveness of emergency plans.

B) Educate the public about disaster risks and preparedness actions.

C) Discourage community participation.

D) Limit the distribution of emergency supplies.

6. Environmental health surveillance is crucial for:

A) Ignoring pollution sources.

B) Tracking the spread of non-communicable diseases.

C) Monitoring environmental conditions and health outcomes.

D) Decreasing public awareness of environmental risks.

7. **A primary goal of antimicrobial stewardship in environmental health is to:**

A) Encourage the misuse of antibiotics.

B) Combat antibiotic resistance.

C) Limit access to necessary medications.

D) Promote the overprescription of treatments.

8. **Community engagement in environmental health efforts is vital for:**

A) Increasing pollution levels.

B) Reducing the sense of community ownership and responsibility.

C) Improving local environmental conditions.

D) Discouraging sustainable practices.

9. **An effective early warning system for disasters provides:**

A) Late warnings about impending disasters.

B) Timely warnings to mitigate the impact of disasters.

C) Confusing messages to the public.

D) No actionable information.

10. **Recovery and rehabilitation after a disaster focus on:**

A) Only short-term emergency relief.

B) Long-term rebuilding and improvements.

C) Ignoring lessons learned from the disaster.

D) Avoiding policy development for future preparedness.

Answers:

1. C) Infectious diseases.

2. B) Regulation and policy enforcement.

3. A) Identifying potential hazards and assessing risks.

4. C) Immediate reconstruction of infrastructure.

5. B) Educate the public about disaster risks and preparedness actions.

6. C) Monitoring environmental conditions and health outcomes.

7. B) Combat antibiotic resistance.

8. C) Improving local environmental conditions.

9. B) Timely warnings to mitigate the impact of disasters.

10. B) Long-term rebuilding and improvements.

Chapter 9: Health Education and Communication

9.1 Effective Health Communication Strategies

Effective health communication is vital for promoting public health, influencing health behaviors, and improving health outcomes. It involves the strategic use of various communication channels to convey health-related information in a manner that is accessible, understandable, and actionable. This subchapter outlines the key strategies for effective health communication, emphasizing the importance of tailoring messages to diverse audiences and utilizing multiple platforms to maximize impact.

Understand Your Audience

- **Audience Segmentation:** Identify and understand the different segments of your target audience based on demographics, health behaviors, cultural backgrounds, and information needs.

- **Cultural Competence:** Ensure messages are culturally relevant and sensitive, respecting the beliefs, practices, and norms of different communities.

Message Development and Framing

- **Clear and Concise Messages:** Develop messages that are straightforward and easy to understand, avoiding medical jargon.

- **Positive Framing:** Focus on the benefits of engaging in healthy behaviors rather than the consequences of unhealthy behaviors.

- **Call to Action:** Include specific, actionable steps that the audience can take to improve their health or access health services.

Utilizing Multiple Channels

- **Diverse Media Platforms:** Leverage a mix of traditional (e.g., radio, television, print materials) and digital media (e.g., social media, websites, mobile apps) to reach broader audiences.

- **Community Engagement:** Use community-based approaches, such as workshops, health fairs, and community meetings, to foster personal connections and engage directly with audiences.

Feedback and Participation

- **Interactive Communication:** Encourage feedback and participation from the audience to create a two-way communication flow, enhancing message relevance and effectiveness.

- **Involvement of Health Professionals:** Engage healthcare providers in communication efforts to add credibility and address audience questions and concerns accurately.

Consistency and Repetition

- **Consistent Messaging:** Ensure that health messages are consistent across different channels and over time to reinforce key points and increase message retention.

- **Regular Updates:** Keep the audience informed with regular updates, especially during health crises or when new health information emerges.

Evaluation and Adaptation

- **Monitoring and Evaluation:** Regularly assess the effectiveness of communication strategies through audience feedback, engagement metrics, and behavior change indicators.

- **Adaptation:** Be prepared to adapt messages and strategies based on evaluation findings and changing health information or audience needs.

Effective health communication is a dynamic and ongoing process that requires careful planning, execution, and evaluation. By implementing these strategies, public health professionals can enhance the clarity, relevance, and impact of health messages, ultimately contributing to improved health literacy, behavior change, and public health outcomes.

9.2 Using Technology in Health Education

The integration of technology into health education has revolutionized the way information is disseminated and how individuals engage with health-related content. Technology offers innovative platforms and tools that can enhance learning, improve access to health information, and foster interactive communication between healthcare providers and the public. This subchapter explores the role of technology in health education, highlighting various applications and their impact on public health initiatives.

Digital Platforms for Information Dissemination

Websites, social media, and mobile apps have become primary sources for health information. These platforms allow health organizations to reach wide audiences, providing timely and accurate health advice, disease outbreak updates, and public health recommendations. Interactive features, such as Q&A sessions, live broadcasts, and discussion forums, further engage users in their health education.

E-Learning and Online Courses

E-learning platforms and online courses offer accessible educational opportunities for both healthcare professionals and the general public. These resources can cover a broad range of topics, from basic health knowledge to specialized medical training. The flexibility of online learning accommodates different learning styles and schedules, making health education more accessible to a wider audience.

Mobile Health (mHealth) Applications

mHealth applications on smartphones and tablets provide tools for health monitoring, disease management, and health promotion. Apps can track physical activity, dietary intake, medication adherence, and more, offering personalized feedback and educational content to users. They can also facilitate remote consultations and health coaching, bridging gaps in healthcare access.

Telehealth and Telemedicine

Telehealth platforms extend educational opportunities by connecting patients with healthcare providers through video conferencing, messaging, and remote monitoring technologies. This direct communication allows for real-time health education, advice, and support, especially beneficial for individuals in remote or underserved areas.

Wearable Technology and Health Monitors

Wearable devices, such as fitness trackers and smartwatches, collect data on physical activity, sleep patterns, and vital signs. These devices not only provide individuals with insights into their health status but can also deliver targeted health education messages and reminders, encouraging healthier lifestyle choices.

Games and Simulations for Health Education

Educational games and simulations engage users in interactive learning experiences, simulating health scenarios or challenges. These tools can be particularly effective in teaching children and young adults about health topics, encouraging engagement and retention of information.

Challenges and Considerations

While technology offers significant benefits for health education, challenges such as digital literacy, privacy concerns, and information accuracy must be addressed. Ensuring content is evidence-based, user-friendly, and accessible to diverse populations is essential for maximizing the impact of technology in health education.

The use of technology in health education represents a promising avenue for enhancing public health knowledge and behaviors. By leveraging digital tools and platforms, health organizations can provide engaging, accessible, and personalized health education, empowering individuals to make informed health decisions and adopt healthier lifestyles.

9.3 Cultural Sensitivity in Health Messaging

Cultural sensitivity in health messaging is crucial for ensuring that health education and communication efforts are effective across diverse populations. Culturally sensitive health messages take into account the beliefs, practices, language, and values of different cultural groups. This approach not only enhances the relevance and acceptability of health information but also increases engagement and adherence to public health recommendations. This subchapter explores the importance of cultural sensitivity in health messaging and strategies for creating inclusive health communications.

Understanding Cultural Contexts

Cultural contexts significantly influence how individuals perceive health and illness, make decisions about healthcare, and engage with health messages. Understanding these contexts involves research and engagement with the target communities to grasp their health beliefs, communication norms, and barriers to health information or services.

Inclusive Language and Representation

Using inclusive language that resonates with the cultural experiences of the target audience is essential. Health messages should avoid medical jargon and be translated into the primary languages spoken by the community. Additionally, visual and multimedia content should reflect the diversity of the community, including representation in terms of race, ethnicity, age, and gender.

Engaging with Community Leaders and Stakeholders

Collaborating with community leaders, healthcare providers, and stakeholders who are respected within the community can enhance the credibility and reach of health messages. These individuals can act as cultural brokers, offering insights into effective communication strategies and helping to tailor messages that are culturally appropriate.

Addressing Health Literacy

Cultural sensitivity also involves considering the varying levels of health literacy within a community. Simplifying complex health information and using clear, accessible formats can help ensure that all members of the community can understand and act upon health messages.

Incorporating Cultural Practices and Values

Incorporating cultural practices, traditions, and values into health messaging can make health education more relevant and engaging. For example, dietary recommendations can be adapted to include culturally specific foods, or physical activity messages can highlight traditional forms of dance or exercise.

Responsive and Adaptive Messaging

Cultural sensitivity requires flexibility and responsiveness to the changing dynamics within communities. Health messaging should be regularly evaluated and adapted based on feedback from the community and emerging cultural trends.

Ethical Considerations

Culturally sensitive health messaging should respect the dignity and autonomy of individuals and communities. It should avoid stereotypes and assumptions, focusing instead on empowering communities with knowledge and choices about their health.

Cultural sensitivity in health messaging is a fundamental component of effective health communication strategies. By recognizing and addressing the diverse cultural contexts of target audiences, health organizations can develop more impactful and engaging health education efforts. This approach not only improves the accessibility of health information but also supports the broader goals of equity and inclusiveness in public health.

9.4 Exercise: 10 MCQs with Answers at the End

Let's craft a set of multiple-choice questions (MCQs) that reflect an understanding of Chapter 9's themes, including effective health communication strategies, the use of technology in health education, and the importance of cultural sensitivity in health messaging. This exercise will help reinforce the key concepts discussed.

1. **Effective health communication strategies should:**

   A) Target a generic audience for simplicity.

   B) Use complex medical jargon to ensure accuracy.

   C) Be tailored to the specific needs and understanding of the audience.

D) Focus exclusively on negative outcomes to motivate change.

2. Which is NOT a benefit of using technology in health education?

A) Provides access to information in remote areas.

B) Allows for personalized health tracking and feedback.

C) Limits the reach of health education to only those with internet access.

D) Offers interactive and engaging learning opportunities.

3. Cultural sensitivity in health messaging is important because it:

A) Guarantees the financial success of health programs.

B) Ensures that messages are ignored by the community.

C) Helps in creating messages that resonate with diverse audiences.

D) Discourages community participation in health initiatives.

4. An example of culturally sensitive health messaging includes:

A) Using a one-size-fits-all approach in all communications.

B) Ignoring the cultural practices and languages of the target audience.

C) Adapting dietary recommendations to include culturally specific foods.

D) Avoiding the use of visual content to prevent misinterpretation.

5. A key strategy for effective health communication is to:

A) Disregard feedback from the target audience.

B) Use fear-based tactics in all health messages.

C) Engage with community leaders and stakeholders.

D) Focus solely on written forms of communication.

6. Mobile health (mHealth) applications can:

A) Only be used for fitness tracking.

B) Provide tools for health monitoring, disease management, and health promotion.

C) Decrease access to health information.

D) Replace traditional healthcare services entirely.

7. Which approach enhances the credibility and reach of health messages?

A) Avoiding collaboration with any community members.

B) Collaborating with community leaders and healthcare providers.

C) Using highly technical language to describe health issues.

D) Limiting messages to only one communication channel.

8. In addressing health literacy, it's important to:

A) Use complex medical terms without explanation.

B) Assume all audience members have a high level of health knowledge.

C) Simplify complex health information into clear, accessible formats.

D) Avoid visual aids as they can confuse the message.

9. Telehealth and telemedicine improve health education by:

A) Limiting patient interaction with healthcare providers.

B) Providing a platform for real-time education, advice, and support.

C) Reducing the need for digital literacy.

D) Encouraging self-diagnosis without professional consultation.

10. A challenge in using technology for health education is:

A) Its ability to reach a wide and diverse audience.

B) The potential for enhancing interactive learning.

C) Addressing digital literacy and privacy concerns.

D) The ease of updating content to reflect the latest health guidelines.

Answers:

1. C) Be tailored to the specific needs and understanding of the audience.

2. C) Limits the reach of health education to only those with internet access.

3. C) Helps in creating messages that resonate with diverse audiences.

4. C) Adapting dietary recommendations to include culturally specific foods.

5. C) Engage with community leaders and stakeholders.

6. B) Provide tools for health monitoring, disease management, and health promotion.

7. B) Collaborating with community leaders and healthcare providers.

8. C) Simplify complex health information into clear, accessible formats.

9. B) Providing a platform for real-time education, advice, and support.

10. C) Addressing digital literacy and privacy concerns.

Chapter 10: Community Mobilization and Engagement

10.1 Principles of Community Mobilization

Community mobilization is a strategic process that engages and motivates a broad sector of the community to take collective action toward a common goal, often related to public health, social issues, or community development. It involves empowering individuals and groups to participate in decision-making processes, contributing to sustainable changes in policies, practices, and social norms. This subchapter outlines the key principles guiding effective community mobilization efforts, highlighting their importance in fostering active community engagement and achieving desired health outcomes.

Participation and Inclusivity

Successful community mobilization relies on the active participation of community members, including traditionally marginalized groups. Inclusivity ensures that diverse perspectives are considered, and everyone has a stake in the outcome, enhancing the relevance and acceptance of initiatives.

Empowerment

Empowerment is a central principle of community mobilization, involving the process of equipping community members with the knowledge, skills, and confidence needed to effect change. Empowerment enables individuals to take control over their health and well-being and advocate for their rights and needs.

Ownership

For community mobilization efforts to be sustainable, the community must take ownership of the process and outcomes. Ownership fosters a sense of responsibility and commitment among community members, ensuring that initiatives continue beyond the life of specific programs.

Partnerships and Collaboration

Building partnerships between community members, local organizations, health agencies, and other stakeholders is crucial. Collaboration leverages the strengths and resources of various groups, facilitating comprehensive approaches to address complex health and social issues.

Capacity Building

Strengthening the capabilities of individuals, organizations, and systems within the community is essential for effective mobilization. Capacity building activities may include training, technical assistance, and resource allocation, supporting the community's ability to plan, implement, and sustain initiatives.

Cultural Sensitivity

Approaches to community mobilization must be culturally sensitive, respecting and integrating the values, beliefs, and customs of the community. Understanding cultural dynamics ensures that efforts are appropriate and effective in engaging community members.

Transparency and Accountability

Maintaining transparency in processes, decisions, and resource allocation is vital for building and maintaining trust with community members. Accountability mechanisms should be established to ensure that commitments are met and community members can provide feedback and hold leaders and organizations responsible.

Adaptability and Flexibility

Community mobilization efforts should be adaptable to changing circumstances and community needs. Flexibility allows initiatives to evolve based on ongoing assessment and feedback, ensuring relevance and effectiveness.

Evidence-Based Approaches

Integrating evidence-based practices and data-driven decision-making into community mobilization enhances the likelihood of success. Using proven strategies and continuously evaluating outcomes inform adjustments and improvements in initiatives.

The principles of community mobilization serve as a foundation for engaging communities in meaningful ways, fostering collaboration, and achieving lasting health and social improvements. By adhering to these principles, community mobilization efforts can effectively address public health challenges, empower individuals and groups, and build resilient and healthy communities.

10.2 Building Community Partnerships for Health

Building community partnerships for health involves the collaboration between individuals, groups, organizations, and sectors to address health issues and promote well-being within communities. These partnerships leverage the unique strengths, resources, and expertise of each partner to implement comprehensive and effective health interventions. This subchapter outlines the strategies for building and sustaining successful community partnerships for health, emphasizing the importance of collective action in achieving health goals.

Identifying and Engaging Stakeholders

The first step in building community partnerships is to identify and engage key stakeholders who have an interest or stake in the health issue being addressed. Stakeholders may include community members, local health providers, non-profit organizations, businesses, schools, and government agencies. Effective engagement involves reaching out to these groups, understanding their perspectives, and inviting their participation.

Establishing Common Goals

Successful partnerships are built on a foundation of shared goals and objectives. Partners should come together to identify common health priorities based on community needs and agree on clear, achievable goals. This collaborative goal-setting process ensures that all partners are aligned and committed to the partnership's success.

Defining Roles and Responsibilities

Clear delineation of roles and responsibilities is crucial for the smooth operation of community partnerships. Each partner should understand their contribution to the partnership, including specific tasks, resource allocation, and timelines. Defining roles and responsibilities helps to prevent overlap, ensure accountability, and facilitate efficient collaboration.

Building Trust and Mutual Respect

Trust and mutual respect are the cornerstones of effective partnerships. These values are cultivated through open communication, transparency in decision-making, and recognition of each partner's contributions. Building trust takes time and requires ongoing effort to maintain.

Developing a Framework for Collaboration

Creating a formal framework for collaboration, such as a memorandum of understanding (MOU) or partnership agreement, can help solidify the partnership. This framework should outline the partnership's structure, governance, decision-making processes, and mechanisms for conflict resolution.

Leveraging Community Assets and Resources

Effective community partnerships identify and utilize the assets and resources available within the community. Asset mapping can reveal a wide range of resources, from physical spaces to the skills and knowledge of community members. Leveraging these assets can enhance the partnership's capacity to implement health initiatives.

Fostering Open Communication

Open and effective communication is essential for the success of community partnerships. Regular meetings, updates, and feedback mechanisms ensure that all partners are informed and engaged. Communication tools and strategies should be accessible and appropriate for the audience.

Evaluating and Celebrating Success

Ongoing evaluation of the partnership's activities and outcomes is important for measuring success and identifying areas for improvement. Celebrating achievements, no matter how small, can motivate partners and reinforce the value of the collaboration.

Sustaining Partnerships

Sustaining community partnerships over the long term requires commitment, flexibility, and adaptation to changing circumstances and needs. Continual efforts to engage new partners, secure resources, and innovate can keep the partnership dynamic and relevant.

Building community partnerships for health is a powerful strategy for addressing complex health challenges. By working collaboratively, leveraging diverse resources, and focusing on shared goals, partnerships can achieve significant and sustainable improvements in community health.

10.3 Volunteerism in Health Care Delivery

Volunteerism plays a pivotal role in health care delivery, particularly in underserved and low-resource settings. Volunteers contribute their time, skills, and enthusiasm to support health services, education, and outreach efforts, often filling gaps in health care provision and enhancing the quality and reach of health services. This subchapter explores the importance of volunteerism in health care delivery, the various roles volunteers play, and strategies for effectively integrating volunteers into health care initiatives.

Importance of Volunteerism in Health Care

Volunteers augment the workforce in health care settings, providing essential services that might otherwise be unavailable due to staffing or resource constraints. They can make health care more accessible, extend services to remote or marginalized communities, and add a valuable human touch to health care delivery. Additionally, volunteerism promotes community engagement and ownership of health care initiatives, strengthening the relationship between health services and the communities they serve.

Roles of Volunteers in Health Care

Volunteers can serve in a variety of roles, depending on their skills, interests, and the needs of the community. Common roles include:

- **Community Health Workers:** Volunteers often serve as community health workers, offering basic health services, education, and referrals in their communities.

- **Support Services:** Volunteers may assist with administrative tasks, patient transport, meal preparation, and other support services in health care facilities.

- **Health Education and Promotion:** Many volunteers engage in health education campaigns, workshops, and outreach programs to raise awareness about health issues and promote healthy behaviors.

- **Advocacy and Fundraising:** Volunteers can act as advocates for health causes, helping to raise awareness and funds for health care programs and research.

Integrating Volunteers into Health Care Delivery

To effectively integrate volunteers into health care delivery, organizations should consider the following strategies:

- **Needs Assessment:** Assess the health care needs of the community and the capacity of existing services to identify areas where volunteers can make a meaningful contribution.

- **Recruitment and Training:** Recruit volunteers based on specific skills and interests, and provide comprehensive training to prepare them for their roles. Ongoing training and support are crucial for volunteer retention and effectiveness.

- **Supervision and Support:** Assign experienced staff to supervise and support volunteers, ensuring they have the guidance and resources needed to perform their duties.

- **Recognition and Appreciation:** Acknowledge the contributions of volunteers through recognition programs, awards, and expressions of appreciation to motivate and retain volunteers.

Challenges and Considerations

While volunteerism adds significant value to health care delivery, it also presents challenges. These include ensuring the quality of services provided by volunteers, maintaining their motivation and commitment, and addressing the ethical implications of volunteer involvement in health care. Clear policies, ethical guidelines, and support systems can help mitigate these challenges.

Impact of Volunteerism on Volunteers and Communities

Volunteerism not only benefits health care delivery but also enriches the lives of volunteers. It provides opportunities for personal growth, skill development, and a sense of purpose and satisfaction from helping others. For communities, volunteerism strengthens social cohesion, promotes a culture of altruism, and empowers community members to take an active role in improving their own health and well-being.

Volunteerism in health care delivery represents a powerful mechanism for enhancing access to care, enriching the patient experience, and building stronger, healthier communities. By leveraging the passion and capabilities of volunteers, health care organizations can extend their reach and impact, making a significant difference in the lives of those they serve.

10.4 Exercise: 10 MCQs with Answers at the End

Creating a set of multiple-choice questions (MCQs) based on Chapter 10, focusing on community mobilization and engagement, including the principles of community mobilization, building community partnerships for health, volunteerism in health care delivery, and their implications for public health, can help consolidate understanding and facilitate learning. Here's a set of MCQs with answers provided:

1. **Effective community mobilization should prioritize:**

   A) Top-down decision-making.

 B) Inclusivity and participation of diverse community members.

   C) Excluding marginalized groups to simplify processes.

   D) Ignoring local cultural practices.

2. **A key benefit of building community partnerships for health is:**

   A) Decreasing community resources.

   B) Reducing the diversity of perspectives in decision-making.

   C) Leveraging the strengths and resources of various stakeholders.

   D) Limiting community involvement in health initiatives.

3. **Volunteers in health care delivery:**

   A) Only provide medical care.

   B) Cannot contribute to health education and promotion.

   C) Play a variety of roles, including support services and health advocacy.

   D) Reduce the quality of health care services.

4. **Which is NOT a principle of community mobilization?**

A) Empowerment.

B) Exclusivity.

C) Ownership.

D) Collaboration.

5. **Effective integration of volunteers into health care delivery requires:**

A) Avoiding training and supervision.

B) Comprehensive training and ongoing support.

C) Discouraging volunteers from interacting with the community.

D) Assigning tasks without considering volunteers' skills and interests.

6. **In building community partnerships for health, defining roles and responsibilities is important to:**

A) Confuse partnership members.

B) Ensure accountability and prevent task overlap.

C) Discourage new members from joining.

D) Limit the scope of the partnership's activities.

7. **Cultural sensitivity in community health initiatives is crucial for:**

A) Undermining community traditions and practices.

B) Creating generic, one-size-fits-all programs.

C) Ensuring relevance and effectiveness of health interventions.

D) Reducing community participation.

8. **A major challenge in volunteerism in health care delivery is:**

A) The overwhelming financial compensation demanded by volunteers.

B) Maintaining the motivation and commitment of volunteers.

C) Having too many volunteers available.

D) Volunteers completely replacing professional health care workers.

9. **Community partnerships for health often involve collaboration between:**

A) Only healthcare professionals.

B) Community members, local organizations, health agencies, and businesses.

C) Competing health care facilities exclusively.

D) Individuals with no interest in health.

10. **Recognition and appreciation of volunteers in health care:**

A) Decreases their motivation.

B) Is unnecessary and has no impact on retention.

C) Can motivate and help retain volunteers.

D) Should be avoided to maintain professional boundaries.

Answers:

1. B) Inclusivity and participation of diverse community members.

2. C) Leveraging the strengths and resources of various stakeholders.

3. C) Play a variety of roles, including support services and health advocacy.

4. B) Exclusivity.

5. B) Comprehensive training and ongoing support.

6. B) Ensure accountability and prevent task overlap.

7. C) Ensuring relevance and effectiveness of health interventions.

8. B) Maintaining the motivation and commitment of volunteers.

9. B) Community members, local organizations, health agencies, and businesses.

10. C) Can motivate and help retain volunteers.

Chapter 11: Health Systems and Policies

11.1 Navigating Health Systems

Navigating health systems involves understanding how healthcare services are organized, financed, and delivered within a community or country. Health systems can vary widely in terms of structure, access, and quality, impacting individuals' ability to receive timely, affordable, and effective care. This subchapter outlines the key components of health systems, challenges individuals may face in accessing care, and strategies for effectively navigating these systems to improve health outcomes.

Key Components of Health Systems

Health systems typically comprise several interrelated components that work together to meet the health needs of the population:

- **Healthcare Providers:** Includes doctors, nurses, specialists, and other healthcare professionals who deliver care.

- **Facilities:** Hospitals, clinics, and other settings where healthcare is provided.

- **Financing:** Mechanisms for funding healthcare, such as insurance, government programs, and out-of-pocket payments.

- **Regulations and Policies:** Guidelines and laws that govern the operation of the health system and the delivery of care.

- **Health Information Systems:** Databases and other tools used to collect, analyze, and communicate health-related information.

Challenges in Navigating Health Systems

Individuals may encounter various obstacles when trying to access healthcare services, including:

- **Complexity:** Health systems can be complex and difficult to understand, especially for those with limited healthcare knowledge or literacy.

- **Cost:** Financial barriers, including high out-of-pocket expenses and lack of insurance coverage, can limit access to care.

- **Availability:** There may be shortages of healthcare providers or facilities, particularly in rural or underserved areas.

- **Quality:** Variability in the quality of care can affect health outcomes and patient satisfaction.

Strategies for Navigating Health Systems

Improving access to and navigation of health systems requires a multifaceted approach:

- **Health Literacy:** Enhancing health literacy helps individuals understand their health needs and the healthcare system, empowering them to make informed decisions.

- **Patient Advocacy:** Advocates can assist individuals in navigating the health system, accessing services, and understanding their rights and options.

- **Integrated Care:** Models of care that integrate services across providers and settings can simplify the healthcare journey for patients, improving coordination and outcomes.

- **Technology:** Digital tools, such as online portals and mobile apps, can provide individuals with easy access to health information, appointment scheduling, and communication with healthcare providers.

- **Policy Reforms:** Reforms aimed at simplifying healthcare access, reducing costs, and improving quality are essential for making health systems more navigable and equitable.

The Role of Health Insurance

Understanding health insurance options, including public, private, and employer-based plans, is crucial for accessing healthcare services. Navigating insurance coverage, benefits, and limitations can help individuals make better-informed decisions about their care and financial responsibilities.

Navigating health systems is a critical skill for achieving optimal health outcomes. By understanding the components and challenges of health systems, individuals can better access the care they need. Efforts to improve health system navigation through education, advocacy, integrated care models, and technology can significantly impact public health and individual well-being.

11.2 The Role of Policy in Community Health

Health policy plays a pivotal role in shaping the health of communities by establishing frameworks for the organization, funding, and delivery of healthcare services. Effective health policies address a wide range of issues, including access to care, quality of healthcare, health disparities, and public health initiatives. This subchapter explores the impact of health policy on community health and strategies for developing and implementing policies that promote the well-being of all community members.

Impact of Health Policy on Community Health

Health policies have a direct impact on the health and well-being of communities. They can:

- **Improve Access to Healthcare:** Policies that provide funding for healthcare services or mandate insurance coverage can make healthcare more accessible to a broader population.

- **Enhance Quality of Care:** Regulations and standards set by health policies ensure that healthcare providers and facilities maintain high levels of quality and safety in patient care.

- **Reduce Health Disparities:** Policies aimed at addressing social determinants of health and providing targeted support to underserved populations can help reduce health disparities.

- **Promote Public Health:** Public health policies that focus on prevention, health promotion, and disease control can improve community health outcomes.

Developing Effective Health Policies

The development of effective health policies involves:

- **Stakeholder Engagement:** Involving a wide range of stakeholders, including healthcare providers, patients, policymakers, and community organizations, in the policy development process ensures that diverse perspectives are considered.

- **Evidence-Based Decision Making:** Utilizing data and research to inform policy decisions helps ensure that policies are grounded in evidence and likely to be effective.

- **Equity Considerations:** Incorporating equity considerations into policy development aims to ensure that policies do not inadvertently exacerbate health disparities.

- **Flexibility and Adaptability:** Policies should be flexible enough to adapt to changing health needs and circumstances.

Implementing Health Policies

Effective implementation of health policies requires:

- **Clear Communication:** Communicating policies clearly to all stakeholders, including healthcare providers, community members, and policymakers, is essential for successful implementation.

- **Adequate Resources:** Ensuring that adequate resources, including funding and personnel, are available to implement policies is crucial.

- **Monitoring and Evaluation:** Continuously monitoring and evaluating the impact of health policies allows for adjustments and improvements to be made over time.

Challenges in Health Policy

Developing and implementing health policies can be challenging due to:

- **Political and Economic Constraints:** Political opposition, economic constraints, and competing priorities can hinder the development and implementation of health policies.

- **Complexity of Health Issues:** The complexity of health issues and the healthcare system can make it difficult to design policies that effectively address all aspects of a problem.

- **Changing Health Needs:** Evolving health needs and emerging health threats require policies to be continuously updated and adapted.

Health policy is a powerful tool for improving community health. By addressing the factors that influence health and healthcare delivery, policies can enhance access to care, improve the quality of services, reduce disparities, and promote the overall well-being of communities. Engaging stakeholders, utilizing evidence-based approaches, and focusing on equity are key strategies for developing and implementing effective health policies.

11.3 Advocacy for Health Policy Change

Advocacy for health policy change is a strategic effort to influence public policies that impact health outcomes and the healthcare system. Advocates work to raise awareness about health issues, mobilize support, and persuade policymakers to enact or modify policies for the betterment of public health. This subchapter discusses the importance of advocacy in shaping health policies, strategies for effective advocacy, and the role of various stakeholders in advocating for health policy change.

Importance of Advocacy in Health Policy

Advocacy plays a crucial role in:

- **Highlighting Public Health Issues:** Advocacy brings attention to critical health issues that may be overlooked or underprioritized by policymakers and the public.

- **Driving Policy Development:** By mobilizing public support and presenting evidence-based solutions, advocacy efforts can lead to the development of new policies or the revision of existing ones.

- **Addressing Health Disparities:** Advocacy focuses on policies that address social determinants of health and aims to reduce health disparities among different population groups.

- **Empowering Communities:** Advocacy empowers communities by giving them a voice in the policy-making process and enabling them to influence decisions that affect their health.

Strategies for Effective Advocacy

Effective health policy advocacy involves several key strategies:

- **Building Coalitions:** Forming coalitions with other organizations and stakeholders strengthens advocacy efforts by pooling resources, expertise, and influence.

- **Utilizing Data and Evidence:** Presenting data and evidence to support policy recommendations makes advocacy efforts more compelling and credible.

- **Engaging Policymakers:** Directly engaging with policymakers through meetings, briefings, and correspondence can influence their understanding and stance on health issues.

- **Mobilizing Public Support:** Generating public support for policy changes through campaigns, petitions, and media outreach can pressure policymakers to act.

- **Leveraging Media and Social Media:** Using traditional media and social media platforms to disseminate messages and rally support broadens the reach and impact of advocacy efforts.

Role of Stakeholders in Advocacy

A wide range of stakeholders can participate in advocacy for health policy change, including:

- **Healthcare Professionals:** Can provide expertise and credibility to advocacy efforts, highlighting the impact of policies on patient care.

- **Non-Governmental Organizations (NGOs):** Often lead advocacy campaigns, utilizing their networks and resources to mobilize support.

- **Community Groups:** Represent the voices and interests of those directly affected by health policies, ensuring that advocacy efforts are grounded in community needs.

- **Individuals:** Patients, families, and concerned citizens can share personal stories and experiences that illustrate the need for policy change.

Challenges in Advocacy

Advocacy efforts can face challenges such as:

- **Political Resistance:** Policymakers may resist changes due to political ideologies, competing interests, or influence from opposing groups.

- **Resource Limitations:** Sustaining advocacy efforts can be resource-intensive, requiring adequate funding, staffing, and expertise.

- **Complexity of Health Policy:** The complexity of health issues and the policy-making process can make it difficult to achieve specific advocacy goals.

Advocacy for health policy change is a powerful mechanism for improving public health outcomes and ensuring that health systems meet the needs of all individuals, especially the most vulnerable. By strategically engaging with stakeholders, utilizing evidence-based arguments, and mobilizing public support, advocates can influence the development and implementation of policies that promote health equity and access to care.

11.4 Exercise: 10 MCQs with Answers at the End

Let's create a set of multiple-choice questions (MCQs) based on Chapter 11, focusing on health systems and policies, including navigating health systems, the role of policy in community health, and advocacy for health policy change. These MCQs aim to test comprehension and reinforce the key concepts discussed.

1. **Navigating health systems effectively requires understanding:**

   A) Only the cost of healthcare services.

   B) The roles of various healthcare providers and facilities.

   C) How to avoid using health insurance.

   D) The benefits of not seeking healthcare.

2. **A key role of health policy in community health is to:**

   A) Increase healthcare costs for patients.

   B) Limit access to quality healthcare services.

   C) Improve access to healthcare and enhance the quality of care.

   D) Discourage public health initiatives.

3. **Effective health policy development should involve:**

A) Ignoring evidence-based research.

B) Solely the opinions of policymakers.

C) Stakeholder engagement and evidence-based decision-making.

D) Decreasing community involvement in health matters.

4. **Health literacy is important for navigating health systems because it:**

A) Limits an individual's ability to make informed health decisions.

B) Helps individuals understand and act upon health information.

C) Is unnecessary for accessing healthcare services.

D) Only benefits healthcare professionals.

5. **Public health policies that focus on prevention and health promotion can:**

A) Worsen community health outcomes.

B) Have no impact on public health.

C) Improve community health outcomes.

D) Only benefit individual health without community impact.

6. **In the context of health policy, equity considerations are important to:**

  A) Ensure policies benefit only certain groups of people.

  B) Address and reduce health disparities.

  C) Increase healthcare costs for underserved populations.

  D) Limit access to healthcare services based on income.

7. **Advocacy for health policy change is essential for:**

  A) Maintaining the status quo in health systems.

  B) Introducing and supporting improvements in healthcare and public health.

  C) Decreasing public engagement in health matters.

  D) Increasing barriers to accessing healthcare.

8. **A major challenge in health policy implementation is:**

  A) The overwhelming support from all political parties.

  B) Adequate funding and resources.

  C) Political and economic constraints.

  D) The simplicity of health issues.

9. **Monitoring and evaluation of health policies are necessary to:**

A) Ensure policies are never updated.

B) Make adjustments and improvements over time.

C) Decrease transparency and accountability.

D) Discourage stakeholder feedback.

10. **Stakeholder engagement in health policy development is crucial because it:**

A) Limits the perspectives considered in policy-making.

B) Ensures that policies are developed in isolation.

C) Incorporates diverse perspectives and strengthens policy relevance.

D) Increases the complexity and confusion in policy-making.

Answers:

1. B) The roles of various healthcare providers and facilities.

2. C) Improve access to healthcare and enhance the quality of care.

3. C) Stakeholder engagement and evidence-based decision-making.

4. B) Helps individuals understand and act upon health information.

5. C) Improve community health outcomes.

6. B) Address and reduce health disparities.

7. B) Introducing and supporting improvements in healthcare and public health.

8. C) Political and economic constraints.

9. B) Make adjustments and improvements over time.

10. C) Incorporates diverse perspectives and strengthens policy relevance.

Chapter 12: Research and Data in Community Health

12.1 Introduction to Health Research Methods

Health research plays a vital role in understanding health issues, evaluating interventions, and informing policy and practice in community health. It involves systematic investigation to establish facts, uncover new knowledge, and develop or test theories and interventions. This subchapter introduces various health research methods used in community health, highlighting their purposes, advantages, and when they are most appropriately applied.

Quantitative Research Methods

Quantitative research involves collecting and analyzing numerical data to understand patterns, relationships, or effects within a population. It is highly structured and uses statistical methods to infer conclusions from the data.

- **Surveys and Questionnaires:** Used to collect data on behaviors, attitudes, or outcomes from a large number of respondents. Useful for assessing health needs, risk factors, and the impact of health interventions.

- **Clinical Trials:** Experimentally test the efficacy of medical interventions, such as drugs or therapies, in controlled settings. They provide strong evidence but can be resource-intensive and complex to conduct.

- **Epidemiological Studies:** Investigate the distribution and determinants of health and disease conditions in specific populations. Include cohort studies, case-control studies, and cross-sectional studies.

Qualitative Research Methods

Qualitative research focuses on understanding the meaning, experiences, and perspectives of participants. It uses non-numerical data and aims to provide depth and context to health issues.

- **Interviews:** In-depth or semi-structured interviews allow for a detailed exploration of individuals' experiences, perceptions, and motivations.

- **Focus Groups:** Group discussions that provide insight into the collective views, norms, and dynamics of a specific group.

- **Ethnography:** Involves immersive observation and participation in communities to understand their cultures, behaviors, and lifestyles in relation to health.

Mixed-Methods Research

Mixed-methods research combines quantitative and qualitative approaches to leverage the strengths of both. It allows for a comprehensive understanding of health issues by quantifying phenomena and exploring the underlying contexts and meanings.

Systematic Reviews and Meta-Analyses

Systematic reviews synthesize findings from multiple studies on a particular health topic, assessing the overall evidence. Meta-analyses statistically combine results from similar studies to derive conclusions about the effect size of an intervention.

Community-Based Participatory Research (CBPR)

CBPR is an approach that actively involves community members in the research process, from defining the research question to disseminating findings. It emphasizes collaboration, empowerment, and capacity building within communities.

Choosing Appropriate Research Methods

Selecting the appropriate research method depends on the research question, the nature of the data, the study population, and the resources available. Each method has its advantages and limitations, and the choice should align with the study's objectives and ethical considerations.

Health research methods are essential tools for advancing knowledge in community health. By employing a variety of research approaches, health professionals and researchers can generate evidence to guide effective interventions, policies, and practices, ultimately improving health outcomes in communities.

12.2 Data Collection and Analysis

Data collection and analysis are fundamental aspects of health research, providing the evidence base for understanding health issues, evaluating interventions, and informing policy decisions. This subchapter delves into the methodologies for collecting and analyzing data in community health research, highlighting best practices and considerations for ensuring reliability and validity.

Data Collection Methods

- **Surveys and Questionnaires:** Widely used for their efficiency in gathering information from a large number of respondents. They can be administered in person, by mail, online, or by telephone. Designing clear and concise questions is crucial for minimizing bias and improving response rates.

- **Interviews:** Can be structured, semi-structured, or unstructured. Interviews allow for in-depth exploration of individual perspectives and experiences. The choice of interview type depends on the research objectives and the level of detail required.

- **Observations:** Direct observation of behaviors, processes, or events in their natural settings provides rich qualitative data. Observational studies can be participant or non-participant, depending on whether researchers engage with the subjects.

- **Biological Samples:** In health research, collecting biological samples (e.g., blood, saliva) can provide objective data on health status, disease markers, or genetic information.

- **Secondary Data Analysis:** Involves analyzing existing data collected for other purposes (e.g., health records, survey data, or registry data). It can be a cost-effective way to conduct research, though researchers must consider the relevance and quality of the data.

Data Analysis Techniques

- **Quantitative Analysis:** Involves statistical methods to summarize, describe, and infer conclusions from numerical data. Techniques vary from basic descriptive statistics to complex inferential models, depending on the research question and design.

- **Qualitative Analysis:** Methods such as thematic analysis, content analysis, or grounded theory are used to interpret patterns, themes, and meanings from textual or observational data. Coding and categorization are essential steps in organizing data for analysis.

- **Mixed-Methods Analysis:** Combines qualitative and quantitative analytical techniques to leverage the strengths of both approaches. It may involve integrating findings in a single study or using one method to build upon or explain findings from the other.

- **Geospatial Analysis:** Uses geographic information system (GIS) technology to analyze and visualize data in relation to physical space. It is particularly useful in epidemiological studies and public health interventions targeting specific geographic areas.

Ensuring Reliability and Validity

- **Reliability:** Refers to the consistency of measurement across time and different observers. Strategies to improve reliability include standardizing data collection procedures and training researchers and interviewers.

- **Validity:** Concerns the accuracy of measurements and the extent to which the methods measure what they are intended to. Validity can be enhanced through careful design of the study and data collection instruments, pilot testing, and the use of established scales and measures.

Ethical Considerations in Data Collection and Analysis

- Ensuring the confidentiality and privacy of participant data is paramount. Researchers must adhere to ethical guidelines, obtain informed consent, and use secure methods for data storage and handling.

- Transparency in data analysis and reporting, including disclosing limitations and potential biases, is essential for the integrity of research.

Effective data collection and analysis are critical for generating valid and reliable findings in community health research. By employing rigorous methods and adhering to ethical standards, researchers can contribute valuable insights to the field of public health.

12.3 Utilizing Data for Health Improvement

The strategic utilization of data plays a crucial role in advancing health improvement initiatives, informing policy decisions, guiding public health interventions, and ultimately enhancing community health outcomes. This subchapter explores how health data can be effectively used to identify health needs, monitor health trends, evaluate the impact of interventions, and support evidence-based decision-making in community health.

Identifying Health Needs and Priorities

Data collected from surveys, health records, and epidemiological studies help to identify the most pressing health needs within a community. Analyzing data on disease prevalence, risk factors, and social determinants of health enables public health officials and community leaders to prioritize interventions that will have the greatest impact on improving health outcomes.

Monitoring Health Trends and Outbreaks

Continuous surveillance and monitoring of health data are essential for detecting emerging health trends, potential outbreaks, and changes in disease patterns. Real-time data analysis can inform timely responses to public health emergencies and guide preventive measures to contain the spread of infectious diseases.

Evaluating the Impact of Health Interventions

Data plays a key role in evaluating the effectiveness of health interventions and programs. By comparing pre- and post-intervention data, researchers can assess changes in health outcomes, behaviors, or risk factors attributable to specific interventions. This evaluation provides valuable feedback on what works, informing the refinement of existing programs and the development of new initiatives.

Supporting Evidence-Based Policy Making

Health data provides the evidence base for developing, implementing, and refining health policies. Policymakers rely on data to make informed decisions about resource allocation, healthcare delivery models, and public health strategies. Data-driven policy making ensures that interventions are targeted, cost-effective, and aligned with community health needs.

Enhancing Community Engagement and Empowerment

Making health data accessible and understandable to community members fosters greater engagement and empowerment in health improvement efforts. Data visualization tools, community health reports, and participatory research approaches can help demystify data, encouraging active participation in health initiatives and advocacy for policy changes.

Leveraging Technology for Data Utilization

Advancements in technology, including electronic health records (EHRs), health information exchanges (HIEs), and mobile health applications, facilitate the collection, analysis, and sharing of health data. These technologies support more integrated, personalized approaches to health care and public health, enabling data-driven decisions at both individual and population levels.

Addressing Data Quality and Equity Issues

Ensuring the quality, accuracy, and representativeness of health data is critical for its effective use in health improvement. Efforts must be made to address data gaps and disparities that may obscure the health needs of marginalized or underserved populations, ensuring that interventions are equitable and inclusive.

Challenges and Considerations

While the utilization of data holds great promise for health improvement, challenges such as data privacy concerns, interoperability issues between different data systems, and the need for data literacy among healthcare providers and the public must be addressed. Ethical considerations in data collection, analysis, and sharing are paramount to maintaining trust and protecting individual rights.

Effectively utilizing data for health improvement requires a collaborative, multi-sectoral approach that values transparency, inclusivity, and ethical standards. By leveraging data to inform actions, community health initiatives can be more strategic, responsive, and impactful, leading to healthier communities and better public health outcomes.

12.4 Exercise: 10 MCQs with Answers at the End

Let's create a set of multiple-choice questions (MCQs) based on Chapter 12, focusing on research and data in community health. This set includes questions on health research methods, data collection and analysis, and utilizing data for health improvement, aiming to reinforce key concepts and insights.

1. **Quantitative research methods in health typically involve:**

   A) Collecting subjective opinions on health issues.

   B) Analyzing non-numerical data like text and images.

   C) Collecting and analyzing numerical data to identify patterns.

D) Conducting in-depth interviews with participants.

2. **A key advantage of qualitative research in health is that it:**

A) Provides statistically significant results.

B) Allows for the exploration of individual experiences and perspectives.

C) Can be generalized to the entire population.

D) Requires less time and resources than quantitative research.

3. **Mixed-methods research combines:**

A) Only surveys and questionnaires.

B) Quantitative and qualitative research approaches.

C) Biological samples with epidemiological studies.

D) Clinical trials with systematic reviews.

4. **In health research, systematic reviews are important because they:**

A) Synthesize findings from a single study.

B) Provide an overview of a topic without analyzing data.

C) Synthesize findings from multiple studies on a particular topic.

D) Offer preliminary data that has not been peer-reviewed.

5. **Effective data collection in community health research requires:**

   A) Using a single method for all types of research questions.

   B) Ignoring ethical considerations to gather more data.

   C) Ensuring the confidentiality and privacy of participant data.

   D) Avoiding the use of technology to maintain data integrity.

6. **Data analysis in health research involves:**

   A) Discarding data that does not support the hypothesis.

   B) Using statistical methods to infer conclusions from numerical data.

   C) Solely relying on researcher intuition to interpret findings.

   D) Exclusively focusing on qualitative data for complex issues.

7. **Utilizing data for health improvement can help:**

   A) Reduce the accuracy of health interventions.

   B) Identify health needs and priorities within a community.

   C) Decrease public health awareness and education efforts.

   D) Limit access to healthcare services based on findings.

8. **Health information systems are crucial for:**

A) Only storing patient medical records.

B) Collecting, analyzing, and communicating health-related information.

C) Reducing the need for data in decision-making processes.

D) Ignoring trends in disease prevalence and risk factors.

9. **Community-based participatory research (CBPR) emphasizes:**

A) The exclusion of community members from the research process.

B) Active involvement of community members in the research process.

C) Sole reliance on external researchers to define the research question.

D) Limiting the dissemination of findings to academic audiences.

10. **In the context of health policy, evidence-based decision-making involves:**

A) Making decisions based on anecdotal evidence and personal opinions.

B) Utilizing data and research to inform policy decisions.

C) Avoiding the use of current research findings in policy development.

D) Relying solely on historical data without considering new evidence.

Answers:

1. C) Collecting and analyzing numerical data to identify patterns.

2. B) Allows for the exploration of individual experiences and perspectives.

3. B) Quantitative and qualitative research approaches.

4. C) Synthesize findings from multiple studies on a particular topic.

5. C) Ensuring the confidentiality and privacy of participant data.

6. B) Using statistical methods to infer conclusions from numerical data.

7. B) Identify health needs and priorities within a community.

8. B) Collecting, analyzing, and communicating health-related information.

9. B) Active involvement of community members in the research process.

10. B) Utilizing data and research to inform policy decisions.

Chapter 13: Emergency Health Response

13.1 Principles of Emergency Health Response

Emergency health response encompasses the actions and strategies employed to protect public health and provide medical care during disasters, outbreaks, and other emergencies. Effective response efforts are crucial for minimizing the health impacts of emergencies, ensuring the continuity of healthcare services, and facilitating recovery. This subchapter outlines the fundamental principles that guide emergency health response, highlighting their significance in orchestrating coordinated, efficient, and effective actions in times of crisis.

Rapid Assessment and Mobilization

- **Quickly assessing the scope and impact of an emergency** is vital to determine the immediate health needs and prioritize response actions. Mobilizing resources, including personnel, equipment, and supplies, in a timely manner is critical for an effective response.

Coordination and Collaboration

- Effective emergency health response requires **coordinated efforts among various stakeholders**, including government agencies, healthcare providers, non-governmental organizations (NGOs), and international bodies. Collaboration ensures a unified approach, avoids duplication of efforts, and leverages the strengths of each participant.

Communication

- **Clear, accurate, and timely communication** with the public, healthcare professionals, and other stakeholders is essential during emergencies. Providing regular updates on the situation, health advisories, and safety measures helps manage public anxiety and ensures compliance with recommended actions.

Adaptability and Flexibility

- Emergencies are dynamic situations that can evolve rapidly. Response efforts must be **adaptable and flexible**, with the ability to adjust plans and strategies based on real-time information and changing conditions.

Equity and Access

- Ensuring **equitable access to healthcare and resources** during emergencies is crucial. Response efforts should address the needs of the most vulnerable populations, including those with pre-existing health conditions, disabilities, the elderly, and marginalized communities.

Sustainability and Capacity Building

- Emergency health responses should consider **long-term sustainability and capacity building**. Strengthening healthcare systems, enhancing preparedness, and investing in training and infrastructure can improve resilience and reduce the impact of future emergencies.

Ethical Considerations

- Adhering to **ethical principles** is paramount in emergency health response. Decisions should be made based on needs, prioritize the welfare of affected populations, and respect the rights and dignity of individuals.

Use of Technology and Innovation

- Leveraging **technology and innovation** can enhance emergency health response. Digital health tools, telemedicine, and data analytics can support surveillance, diagnostics, patient care, and resource management.

Community Engagement

- **Engaging with communities** and understanding their needs, perceptions, and capacities is essential for effective emergency response. Community participation can enhance the relevance and acceptance of response efforts, and support recovery and resilience building.

Health System Strengthening

- A robust emergency health response is underpinned by a strong health system. Efforts to **strengthen health systems** before, during, and after emergencies are essential for maintaining healthcare delivery and improving overall preparedness.

The principles of emergency health response provide a framework for addressing health emergencies comprehensively and effectively. By adhering to these principles, emergency responders can ensure that health interventions are timely, coordinated, and capable of meeting the diverse needs of affected populations, ultimately saving lives and promoting recovery.

13.2 Managing Epidemics and Pandemics

Managing epidemics and pandemics requires a coordinated global and local response to control the spread of infectious diseases and minimize their impact on health, society, and economies. Effective management strategies are critical for containing outbreaks, protecting vulnerable populations, and preventing future health crises. This subchapter outlines key approaches and considerations in managing epidemics and pandemics, emphasizing the importance of preparedness, rapid response, and international cooperation.

Surveillance and Early Detection

- Early detection of infectious disease outbreaks is essential for prompt response and containment. Robust surveillance systems, including laboratory testing, reporting mechanisms, and epidemiological monitoring, help identify outbreaks quickly and track their spread.

Rapid Response and Containment

- Once an outbreak is detected, immediate actions are required to contain it. This may include isolating cases, implementing quarantine measures, conducting contact tracing, and imposing travel restrictions. Rapid response teams play a crucial role in these efforts.

Public Health Interventions

- A range of public health interventions may be employed to control epidemics and pandemics, including social distancing measures, mask-wearing mandates, and hygiene campaigns. Public compliance with these interventions is crucial for their effectiveness.

Vaccination

- Vaccines are a critical tool in preventing and controlling infectious diseases. Accelerating vaccine development, ensuring equitable distribution, and promoting vaccination uptake are key components of pandemic response efforts.

Healthcare System Strengthening

- Epidemics and pandemics place significant strain on healthcare systems. Strengthening healthcare infrastructure, ensuring adequate supplies of medical equipment and protective gear, and supporting healthcare workers are essential for managing increased patient loads and providing care.

International Cooperation

- Infectious diseases do not respect borders, making international cooperation vital for effective epidemic and pandemic management. Sharing information, resources, and best practices can enhance global preparedness and response.

Communication and Public Education

- Clear, accurate, and timely communication with the public is essential during epidemics and pandemics. Public education campaigns can provide crucial information about disease prevention, symptoms, and treatment options, helping to alleviate fear and misinformation.

Research and Development

- Ongoing research and development are critical for understanding infectious diseases and developing new diagnostics, treatments, and vaccines. Collaboration between governments, academia, and the private sector can accelerate these efforts.

Social and Economic Support

- Epidemics and pandemics can have significant social and economic impacts. Providing support to individuals and communities affected by outbreaks, including financial assistance and mental health services, is important for recovery and resilience.

Ethical Considerations

- Managing epidemics and pandemics raises ethical considerations, including balancing individual rights with public health needs and ensuring equitable access to healthcare and resources. Ethical frameworks can guide decision-making during health crises.

Effective management of epidemics and pandemics requires a multifaceted approach that combines public health interventions, healthcare system strengthening, international collaboration, and community engagement. By learning from past outbreaks and investing in preparedness and response capabilities, societies can better navigate the challenges posed by infectious diseases and safeguard public health.

13.3 First Aid and Basic Life Support

First Aid and Basic Life Support (BLS) are crucial components of emergency health response, providing immediate care and support to individuals experiencing a medical emergency or injury until professional medical help arrives. Knowledge and skills in first aid and BLS can save lives, prevent conditions from worsening, and provide critical support in crisis situations. This subchapter delves into the key concepts, techniques, and importance of first aid and basic life support in the context of community health.

First Aid Basics

First aid involves a range of simple medical techniques and practices aimed at assisting individuals who are injured or in immediate need of medical attention. Key aspects of first aid include:

- **Assessment:** Quickly and safely assessing the individual's condition to determine the type of assistance needed.

- **Immediate Care:** Providing immediate care for injuries or conditions, such as controlling bleeding, applying dressings, stabilizing fractures, and addressing burns or wounds.

- **CPR (Cardiopulmonary Resuscitation):** Performing CPR on individuals who are unresponsive and not breathing, to maintain circulation and oxygenation until emergency services arrive.

- **Safety and Prevention:** Ensuring the safety of both the responder and the individual in need, and preventing further harm or injury.

Basic Life Support (BLS) Techniques

BLS is a level of medical care used for victims of life-threatening illnesses or injuries until they can be given full medical care at a hospital. It includes:

- **Airway Management:** Ensuring that the individual's airway is clear and open to facilitate breathing.

- **Breathing Support:** Providing rescue breathing or ventilations to support or restore breathing.

- **Circulation Support:** Using chest compressions to maintain blood circulation in individuals with no pulse.

- **Automated External Defibrillator (AED) Use:** Applying an AED to deliver a shock to an individual experiencing sudden cardiac arrest when appropriate.

Training and Certification

- Receiving training and certification in first aid and BLS is essential for effectively providing care. Many organizations, such as the Red Cross, American Heart Association, and local health departments, offer courses that cover the necessary skills and knowledge.

- Regular refresher courses are recommended to ensure skills remain current and effective.

Importance in Community Health

- Knowledge of first aid and BLS is valuable for everyone, not just healthcare professionals. It empowers community members to act confidently and competently in emergency situations, potentially saving lives.

- Promoting widespread first aid and BLS training within communities enhances overall preparedness for emergencies, reduces the severity of injuries or medical conditions, and improves outcomes.

Ethical and Legal Considerations

- While providing first aid and BLS, individuals should be aware of ethical and legal considerations, including consent and the duty to act within one's level of training. In many regions, Good Samaritan laws offer legal protection to those who provide assistance in good faith.

First aid and basic life support are integral to emergency health response, emphasizing the importance of immediate care in saving lives and minimizing the impact of injuries and acute medical conditions. Encouraging and facilitating training in these critical skills within communities can significantly enhance collective resilience and emergency preparedness.

13.4 Exercise: 10 MCQs with Answers at the End

Creating a set of multiple-choice questions (MCQs) based on Chapter 13, focusing on emergency health response, including principles of emergency health response, managing epidemics and pandemics, first aid, and basic life support, offers a comprehensive review of crucial concepts. Here's a tailored set of MCQs with answers provided:

1. **The initial step in an effective emergency health response is:**

   A) Mobilizing community volunteers.

   B) Rapid assessment of the situation.

C) Distributing medical supplies indiscriminately.

D) Waiting for external aid.

2. **In managing epidemics and pandemics, surveillance and early detection are crucial for:**

A) Ensuring the disease spreads to achieve herd immunity.

B) Identifying outbreaks quickly and tracking their spread.

C) Reducing healthcare costs.

D) Promoting travel to affected areas.

3. **Which is NOT a principle of Basic Life Support (BLS)?**

A) Airway management.

B) Providing immediate financial assistance.

C) Circulation support through chest compressions.

D) Use of Automated External Defibrillator (AED).

4. **During an epidemic, public health interventions might include:**

A) Encouraging large public gatherings.

B) Social distancing measures.

C) Reducing vaccination efforts.

D) Ignoring hygiene practices.

5. **First aid training is important because it:**

A) Is only necessary for medical professionals.

B) Empowers individuals to provide immediate care in emergencies.

C) Should be avoided to prevent legal issues.

D) Is less effective than waiting for professional help.

6. **Which is a key role of international cooperation in managing pandemics?**

A) Withholding information about outbreaks.

B) Competing for medical resources.

C) Sharing surveillance data and resources.

D) Promoting travel between affected countries.

7. **Effective communication in emergency health response involves:**

A) Providing vague and infrequent updates.

B) Clear, accurate, and timely information.

C) Using medical jargon to describe the situation.

D) Discouraging public inquiries.

8. **The use of technology in emergency health response can:**

   A) Increase the time needed to respond to emergencies.

   B) Enhance surveillance, diagnostics, and patient care.

   C) Reduce the accuracy of health data.

   D) Limit communication between responders.

9. **An ethical consideration in providing first aid is:**

   A) Avoiding care to those who cannot pay.

   B) Providing care only to certain demographics.

   C) Acting within one's level of training and obtaining consent.

   D) Refusing to help to avoid legal repercussions.

10. **A major challenge in pandemic management is:**

   A) The overabundance of medical supplies.

   B) Ensuring equitable access to healthcare and resources.

   C) The rapid development of too many effective vaccines.

   D) Decreased public interest in health information.

Answers:

1. B) Rapid assessment of the situation.

2. B) Identifying outbreaks quickly and tracking their spread.

3. B) Providing immediate financial assistance.

4. B) Social distancing measures.

5. B) Empowers individuals to provide immediate care in emergencies.

6. C) Sharing surveillance data and resources.

7. B) Clear, accurate, and timely information.

8. B) Enhance surveillance, diagnostics, and patient care.

9. C) Acting within one's level of training and obtaining consent.

10. B) Ensuring equitable access to healthcare and resources.

Chapter 14: Ethical Considerations in Community Health

14.1 Ethics and Confidentiality

In the field of community health, ethical considerations are paramount to ensuring that health care practices and research uphold the highest standards of integrity and respect for individuals and communities. Among these considerations, confidentiality stands out as a fundamental principle, safeguarding the privacy of personal health information. This subchapter explores the importance of ethics and confidentiality in community health, the challenges faced, and strategies for maintaining confidentiality in various settings.

The Importance of Ethics in Community Health

Ethics in community health encompasses a broad spectrum of considerations, including respect for autonomy, justice, beneficence, and non-maleficence. Ethical practices ensure that individuals and communities receive care and participate in research in a manner that respects their rights, dignity, and values.

Confidentiality as a Core Ethical Principle

Confidentiality involves the obligation of healthcare providers and researchers to protect personal health information from unauthorized access, use, or disclosure. This principle is critical for:

- Building trust between healthcare providers and patients.

- Encouraging individuals to seek care and fully disclose their health status.

- Protecting individuals from potential discrimination or stigma based on their health information.

Challenges in Maintaining Confidentiality

Maintaining confidentiality can be challenging due to:

- The increasing use of electronic health records (EHRs) and health information exchanges (HIEs), which, while improving efficiency and coordination of care, may pose risks to data security.

- The need for information sharing among healthcare providers for coordinated care, which must be balanced with the imperative to protect patient privacy.

- Community health research that requires the collection, analysis, and reporting of health data, necessitating stringent measures to anonymize data and secure informed consent.

Strategies for Upholding Confidentiality

- **Implementing Robust Data Protection Measures:** Utilizing encryption, secure access controls, and regular audits to protect electronic health data.

- **Training Healthcare Providers:** Ensuring that all members of the healthcare team understand their responsibilities regarding confidentiality and are trained in privacy protection practices.

- **Informed Consent in Research:** Clearly communicating the purpose, methods, risks, and benefits of research to participants and obtaining their informed consent, with explicit agreements on how their data will be used and protected.

- **Legislative Compliance:** Adhering to laws and regulations governing health information privacy, such as the Health Insurance Portability and Accountability Act (HIPAA) in the United States.

Ethical Decision-Making

Ethical decision-making in community health often requires navigating complex situations where competing interests and values must be balanced. Frameworks for ethical decision-making can help guide healthcare providers and researchers in making choices that respect confidentiality while fulfilling other ethical obligations.

Ethics and confidentiality are foundational to the practice of community health, ensuring that individuals' rights and privacy are protected while providing high-quality care and conducting vital research. By adhering to ethical principles and implementing effective strategies for maintaining confidentiality, community health professionals can foster trust, promote well-being, and contribute to the overall health of communities.

14.2 Ethical Dilemmas in Health Care Delivery

Ethical dilemmas in health care delivery arise when healthcare professionals face situations requiring them to make difficult choices between competing ethical principles, values, or interests. These dilemmas often involve conflicts between respecting patient autonomy, ensuring beneficence, avoiding non-maleficence, and promoting justice. This subchapter examines common ethical dilemmas encountered in health care delivery and discusses approaches for navigating these complex situations.

Consent and Autonomy vs. Beneficence

One common ethical dilemma occurs when a patient's autonomous decision conflicts with what healthcare professionals consider being in the patient's best interest (beneficence). For example, a patient may refuse a life-saving treatment due to personal or cultural beliefs.

Approach: Healthcare providers must respect patient autonomy while also ensuring that patients are fully informed about the consequences of their decisions. Engaging in open, empathetic communication and seeking to understand the patient's perspective can help find a balance between respecting autonomy and promoting beneficence.

Resource Allocation and Justice

Another dilemma involves allocating limited healthcare resources in a way that is just and equitable. This can be particularly challenging during public health emergencies, where the demand for healthcare services exceeds the available resources.

Approach: Principles of justice require that resources be allocated fairly, based on medical need, and without discrimination. Ethical frameworks, such as prioritizing the most vulnerable or maximizing the number of lives saved, can guide decision-making in these situations.

Confidentiality vs. The Duty to Warn

Healthcare providers may face dilemmas involving the need to maintain patient confidentiality versus the duty to warn others of potential harm. For instance, if a patient discloses information suggesting they pose a risk to someone else's safety, healthcare providers must weigh the importance of confidentiality against the need to prevent harm.

Approach: Navigating this dilemma requires careful consideration of legal obligations, ethical principles, and the potential consequences of action or inaction. Consulting with ethics committees or legal advisors can provide guidance in making these difficult decisions.

End-of-Life Care Decisions

End-of-life care often presents ethical dilemmas related to prolonging life versus respecting a patient's wishes for quality of life and dignity in death. Decisions about withdrawing or withholding life-sustaining treatments can be particularly complex.

Approach: Ethical decision-making in end-of-life care should involve discussions with the patient (if possible), their family, and the healthcare team. Advance care planning and directives can also help ensure that care aligns with the patient's values and wishes.

Navigating Ethical Dilemmas

When facing ethical dilemmas in health care delivery, healthcare professionals can utilize several strategies to navigate these challenges effectively:

- **Ethical Frameworks and Guidelines:** Applying established ethical frameworks and guidelines can help clarify the values at stake and guide decision-making.

- **Interdisciplinary Collaboration:** Consulting with colleagues, ethics committees, and other professionals can provide diverse perspectives and support in resolving dilemmas.

- **Continuous Education:** Ongoing education in medical ethics equips healthcare providers with the knowledge and skills to address ethical challenges competently.

- **Patient and Family Engagement:** Involving patients and their families in discussions and decisions ensures that care respects individual values and preferences.

Ethical dilemmas in health care delivery require thoughtful consideration and a balanced approach to decision-making. By adhering to ethical principles, engaging in open dialogue, and seeking collaborative solutions, healthcare providers can navigate these dilemmas while upholding the integrity and values of the medical profession.

14.3 Consent and Community Rights

In the realm of community health, the principles of consent and the recognition of community rights are essential for ensuring ethical engagement and respecting individual autonomy within the context of public health initiatives. This subchapter explores the nuances of obtaining consent in community health settings, the rights of communities to participate in decisions that affect their well-being, and strategies for balancing individual rights with collective health goals.

Understanding Consent in Community Health

Consent in community health involves obtaining explicit permission from individuals or communities before conducting health interventions, research, or collecting personal health information. It is rooted in the ethical principles of autonomy and respect, allowing individuals and communities to make informed decisions about their participation.

Challenges in Obtaining Consent

- **Cultural and Linguistic Differences:** Variations in languages, literacy levels, and cultural norms can impact the consent process, requiring tailored approaches to ensure understanding and voluntariness.

- **Informed Consent:** Ensuring that consent is truly informed involves clearly explaining the purpose, procedures, risks, benefits, and alternatives of the intervention or research, which can be challenging in complex or emergency situations.

- **Community vs. Individual Consent:** In community-based interventions or research, obtaining consent from entire communities or their representatives poses unique challenges, particularly in defining who has the authority to consent on behalf of the community.

Community Rights in Health Care

Community rights encompass the collective rights of communities to participate in decision-making processes, access health care services equitably, and protect their cultural, social, and environmental determinants of health. Recognizing community rights involves:

- **Participation:** Encouraging active involvement of community members in planning, implementing, and evaluating health programs.

- **Transparency and Accountability:** Ensuring that health initiatives are transparent, with clear communication about goals, processes, and outcomes, and mechanisms for community feedback and accountability.

- **Equity:** Addressing health disparities and ensuring that health interventions do not disproportionately burden vulnerable or marginalized populations.

Balancing Individual Rights and Public Health Goals

Ethical dilemmas often arise when individual rights to autonomy and consent conflict with public health goals aimed at benefiting the wider community. Strategies for navigating these conflicts include:

- **Ethical Frameworks:** Employing ethical frameworks that balance respect for individual autonomy with the principle of beneficence, or doing good for the community.

- **Community Engagement:** Engaging with communities to understand their values, needs, and preferences can help design health interventions that respect individual rights while achieving public health objectives.

- **Negotiated Consent:** In situations where individual informed consent may not be feasible, such as large-scale public health interventions, negotiated consent processes involving community representatives can provide a form of collective consent.

Strategies for Upholding Consent and Community Rights

- **Cultural Competence:** Developing cultural competence among health professionals to effectively communicate and engage with diverse communities.

- **Education and Empowerment:** Educating communities about their health rights and empowering them to participate actively in health decisions.

- **Continuous Dialogue:** Maintaining ongoing dialogue between health authorities and communities to build trust, adjust interventions as needed, and address concerns and preferences.

Consent and community rights are foundational to ethical practice in community health, ensuring that interventions are respectful, culturally sensitive, and aligned with the values and needs of individuals and communities. By prioritizing informed consent, community participation, and the protection of community rights, public health efforts can achieve their goals while upholding ethical standards and fostering trust and cooperation.

14.4 Exercise: 10 MCQs with Answers at the End

Creating a set of multiple-choice questions (MCQs) based on Chapter 14, focusing on ethical considerations in community health, including ethics and confidentiality, ethical dilemmas in health care delivery, consent and community rights, aims to reinforce the understanding of these critical concepts. Here's a tailored set of MCQs with the answers provided:

1. **Confidentiality in community health ensures:**

   A) Information is shared with everyone to promote community awareness.

B) Personal health information is protected from unauthorized access.

C) Healthcare providers can make decisions without patient consent.

D) Community health initiatives are prioritized over individual rights.

2. **An ethical dilemma in health care delivery often arises from:**

A) Clear guidelines that eliminate any form of uncertainty.

B) A situation requiring a choice between competing ethical principles.

C) The straightforward application of community health policies.

D) Avoiding any form of patient interaction to reduce ethical challenges.

3. **Informed consent is crucial for:**

A) Allowing healthcare professionals to bypass patient preferences.

B) Providing patients and communities with control over their health care decisions.

C) Simplifying the research process by eliminating the need for explanations.

D) Reducing the quality of care by overwhelming patients with information.

4. **Community rights in health care primarily involve:**

A) Limiting community involvement in health care decision-making.

B) Participation and transparency in health initiatives that affect the community.

C) Ensuring that communities comply with health authorities without question.

D) Withholding information about health programs to prevent public panic.

5. **Balancing individual rights with public health goals requires:**

A) Ignoring individual rights in favor of collective health benefits.

B) Ethical frameworks that consider both autonomy and beneficence.

C) Solely focusing on individual preferences, regardless of public health impact.

D) The complete elimination of public health interventions.

6. **Ethical considerations in community health include all except:**

A) Ensuring equitable access to health care services.

B) Promoting justice and beneficence in health interventions.

C) Using health data for personal gain of healthcare providers.

D) Respecting patient autonomy and confidentiality.

7. **A key challenge in maintaining confidentiality with electronic health records (EHRs) is:**

A) The ease of manually altering paper records.

B) Enhancing the user-friendliness of health apps.

C) Protecting data against unauthorized access and breaches.

D) Encouraging patients to avoid using EHRs for their health information.

8. **Consent in community health research is particularly challenging due to:**

A) The unanimous agreement on all aspects of research within communities.

B) Cultural and linguistic differences that may affect understanding.

C) The preference for using outdated methods of data collection.

D) Communities' general disinterest in health improvement efforts.

9. **Ethical frameworks in health care help navigate dilemmas by:**

A) Providing rigid rules that apply to all situations without exception.

B) Offering guidelines that balance competing values and interests.

C) Eliminating the need for professional judgment and discretion.

D) Discouraging the consideration of ethical principles in decision-making.

10. Community engagement in ethical health care delivery:

A) Is unnecessary and can hinder the efficiency of health interventions.

B) Plays a crucial role in ensuring interventions are culturally sensitive and accepted.

C) Should be avoided to prevent biases in health care provision.

D) Only benefits health care providers, not the community members.

Answers:

1. B) Personal health information is protected from unauthorized access.

2. B) A situation requiring a choice between competing ethical principles.

3. B) Providing patients and communities with control over their health care decisions.

4. B) Participation and transparency in health initiatives that affect the community.

5. B) Ethical frameworks that consider both autonomy and beneficence.

6. C) Using health data for personal gain of healthcare providers.

7. C) Protecting data against unauthorized access and breaches.

8. B) Cultural and linguistic differences that may affect understanding.

9. B) Offering guidelines that balance competing values and interests.

10. B) Plays a crucial role in ensuring interventions are culturally sensitive and accepted.

Chapter 15: Building a Sustainable Future in Community Health

15.1 Sustainability in Health Initiatives

Sustainability in health initiatives refers to the capacity to maintain health programs and outcomes over the long term, ensuring that the benefits continue to accrue for the community without causing undue harm to resources or the environment. A sustainable approach in community health not only addresses current health challenges but also anticipates future needs, adapting to changes while preserving resources for future generations. This subchapter explores key concepts, strategies, and challenges associated with building sustainability in health initiatives.

Key Concepts of Sustainability in Health

- **Long-term Impact:** Sustainability focuses on creating lasting health improvements that persist beyond the initial period of intervention.

- **Resource Efficiency:** Efficient use of financial, human, and natural resources ensures that health initiatives do not deplete the resources necessary for future health needs.

- **Adaptability:** Sustainable health initiatives are flexible and adaptable to changing health landscapes, including demographic shifts, emerging health threats, and evolving community needs.

Strategies for Enhancing Sustainability

- **Community Engagement and Ownership:** Involving community members in the planning, implementation, and evaluation of health initiatives fosters local ownership and increases the likelihood of sustainability.

- **Capacity Building:** Strengthening the skills and capabilities of local healthcare providers, leaders, and organizations ensures that communities can continue health initiatives independently.

- **Partnerships and Collaboration:** Collaborating with local governments, NGOs, and other stakeholders can pool resources, share knowledge, and build a stronger foundation for sustainable health efforts.

- **Integrated Approaches:** Integrating health initiatives into broader development goals, such as education, economic development, and environmental protection, creates synergies that enhance sustainability.

- **Monitoring and Evaluation:** Continuous monitoring and evaluation allow for adjustments to be made over time, ensuring that health initiatives remain effective and relevant.

Challenges to Sustainability

- **Funding and Resource Constraints:** Securing long-term funding and managing resources efficiently are significant challenges for sustaining health initiatives.

- **Changing Health Needs:** Adapting to shifting health needs and priorities requires ongoing assessment and flexibility, which can be difficult to manage.

- **Environmental Impact:** Ensuring that health initiatives do not adversely affect the environment or deplete natural resources adds complexity to planning and implementation.

Case Studies of Sustainable Health Initiatives

Examples of successful sustainable health initiatives include community-based health insurance schemes that improve access to care while being financially viable, and public health programs that integrate environmental conservation efforts, such as clean water and sanitation projects, which have long-term health benefits.

Moving Forward

Building a sustainable future in community health requires a comprehensive approach that balances immediate health needs with long-term goals, engages communities as active participants, and leverages partnerships for broader impact. By focusing on sustainability, community health initiatives can create enduring improvements in health outcomes, contribute to the resilience of communities, and support the well-being of future generations.

Sustainability in community health is an ongoing journey, necessitating commitment, innovation, and collaboration. As communities and health systems evolve, so too must the approaches to ensuring that health interventions are sustainable, equitable, and effective in the face of changing global health landscapes.

15.2 Innovation and Adaptation in Health Services

Innovation and adaptation are pivotal in the ever-evolving landscape of community health services, enabling the development and implementation of effective, efficient, and responsive health care models. These processes allow health systems to meet current and future challenges, including emerging health threats, changing population needs, and advancements in medical technology. This subchapter discusses the importance of innovation and adaptation in health services, highlighting examples and strategies for fostering a culture of continuous improvement.

Importance of Innovation in Health Services

- **Meeting Emerging Health Needs:** Innovation helps address new or evolving health challenges, such as pandemics, antibiotic resistance, and non-communicable diseases.

- **Enhancing Access and Quality:** Innovative health care models and technologies can improve access to care, especially in underserved areas, and enhance the quality and efficiency of health services.

- **Cost-Effectiveness:** New approaches can streamline operations and reduce costs, making health systems more sustainable in the long term.

Examples of Innovation in Health Services

- **Telemedicine and Digital Health:** The use of digital platforms for remote consultations, monitoring, and health information exchange has transformed access to care, making it more convenient and accessible.

- **Mobile Health (mHealth) Applications:** Apps that promote healthy behaviors, disease management, and patient education empower individuals to take an active role in their health care.

- **Point-of-Care Diagnostics:** Portable and easy-to-use diagnostic tools enable rapid, on-site health assessments, crucial for early detection and management of diseases.

Adaptation in Health Services

Adaptation involves modifying health services to respond to changing conditions and needs. It encompasses not only the adoption of new technologies and practices but also the reevaluation and modification of existing services.

Strategies for Fostering Innovation and Adaptation

- **Encouraging a Culture of Learning:** Creating an environment that values continuous learning, experimentation, and feedback encourages innovation and allows for the rapid adaptation of successful practices.

- **Collaborative Partnerships:** Engaging in partnerships with academic institutions, technology companies, and other sectors can bring fresh perspectives and resources to health service innovation.

- **Community Involvement:** Involving community members in the design and implementation of health services ensures that innovations are relevant, culturally appropriate, and more likely to be adopted.

- **Policy Support and Funding:** Governments and organizations can support innovation through policies that encourage research and development, provide funding for pilot projects, and create regulatory environments that foster the adoption of new technologies.

Challenges to Innovation and Adaptation

- **Resistance to Change:** Institutional and individual resistance can hinder the adoption of new practices and technologies.

- **Resource Limitations:** Limited funding and resources can restrict the ability to develop and implement innovative solutions.

- **Ensuring Equity:** It's essential to ensure that innovations in health services are accessible to all segments of the population, including the most vulnerable.

Moving Forward

As community health services continue to evolve, fostering a culture of innovation and adaptation will be critical for addressing the complex health challenges of the 21st century. By embracing change, encouraging creativity, and leveraging new technologies, health services can improve outcomes, enhance patient experiences, and build stronger, healthier communities.

15.3 Fostering Resilience in Communities

Fostering resilience in communities involves strengthening their capacity to anticipate, prepare for, respond to, and recover from health challenges and adversities. A resilient community can effectively navigate the complexities of public health emergencies, environmental changes, and social disparities, ensuring sustainable health and well-being for its members. This subchapter explores strategies and principles for building community resilience in the context of health.

Key Components of Community Resilience

- **Social Cohesion and Connectivity:** Strong social networks and connections within a community enhance mutual support, information sharing, and collective action in times of crisis.

- **Local Knowledge and Participation:** Leveraging local knowledge and encouraging active community participation in health planning and decision-making empower communities to address their unique health challenges.

- **Economic Stability:** Economic stability and access to resources are fundamental for ensuring that communities can invest in health infrastructure, services, and recovery efforts.

- **Adaptive Capacity:** The ability of a community to adapt to changing health landscapes, including emerging threats and opportunities, is crucial for long-term resilience.

- **Integrated Health Services:** A resilient community health system is integrated, accessible, and capable of meeting diverse health needs, including during emergencies.

Strategies for Fostering Community Resilience

- **Community-Based Health Planning:** Involving community members in health planning processes ensures that interventions are culturally appropriate, targeted, and more likely to be sustainable.

- **Education and Capacity Building:** Providing education on health risks and resilience-building practices, along with training community health workers and volunteers, strengthens community-wide health literacy and response capabilities.

- **Infrastructure Development:** Investing in resilient health infrastructure, including facilities, technologies, and supply chains, ensures continuity of care and services during disasters.

- **Environmental Sustainability:** Promoting environmental sustainability practices helps protect communities from health impacts related to environmental degradation and climate change.

- **Psychosocial Support:** Providing psychosocial support and mental health services helps individuals and communities cope with and recover from the psychological impacts of health emergencies and adversities.

Challenges in Building Community Resilience

- **Resource Limitations:** Limited financial and human resources can constrain resilience-building efforts, particularly in low-resource settings.

- **Inequities and Disparities:** Existing social and health inequities can undermine resilience, requiring targeted efforts to address the needs of the most vulnerable populations.

- **Coordination and Collaboration:** Effective collaboration between community groups, health agencies, government bodies, and other stakeholders is necessary but can be challenging to achieve.

Case Studies of Resilient Communities

Successful examples of community resilience often involve multi-sectoral collaboration, innovative use of local resources, and strong leadership. These case studies highlight the importance of tailored, context-specific approaches to resilience-building.

Moving Forward

Fostering resilience in communities is a dynamic and ongoing process. It requires a holistic approach that addresses health, social, economic, and environmental factors. By prioritizing resilience-building, communities can enhance their capacity to withstand and recover from health challenges, contributing to a sustainable future in community health. Engaging communities, leveraging local strengths, and ensuring equitable access to resources and opportunities are key strategies for building resilient communities capable of navigating the complexities of modern public health challenges.

15.4 Exercise: 10 MCQs with Answers at the End

Creating a set of multiple-choice questions (MCQs) based on Chapter 15, focusing on building a sustainable future in community health, including sustainability in health initiatives, innovation and adaptation in health services, and fostering community resilience, can help encapsulate the core concepts and facilitate learning. Here's a tailored set of MCQs with the answers provided:

1. **Sustainability in health initiatives primarily aims to:**

   A) Focus solely on short-term health outcomes.

   B) Ensure long-term health benefits and resource conservation.

   C) Increase dependency on external funding and support.

   D) Isolate health initiatives from broader community development efforts.

2. **Which of the following is a key component of community resilience?**

   A) Social isolation

   B) Economic instability

   C) Adaptive capacity

   D) Centralized decision-making

3. **Innovation in health services often involves:**

A) Avoiding the use of technology in healthcare.

B) Implementing proven traditional methods without modifications.

C) Introducing new models or technologies to improve care.

D) Strictly adhering to past practices regardless of outcomes.

4. **Which strategy is NOT effective for fostering resilience in communities?**

A) Enhancing economic stability

B) Promoting environmental sustainability

C) Discouraging community participation in health planning

D) Investing in psychosocial support and mental health services

5. **A challenge in maintaining sustainability in health initiatives is:**

A) The consistent overabundance of resources.

B) Adapting to changing health needs and priorities.

C) The universal acceptance of new health interventions by all community members.

D) The automatic integration of health initiatives into community development.

6. Telemedicine and digital health innovations aim to:

A) Reduce access to healthcare services.

B) Limit patient autonomy and control over health decisions.

C) Improve access to care and the efficiency of health services.

D) Increase the cost of health care delivery.

7. Economic stability contributes to community resilience by:

A) Decreasing the community's capacity to invest in health initiatives.

B) Increasing dependency on external aid.

C) Ensuring communities have resources for health infrastructure and services.

D) Encouraging the neglect of long-term health planning.

8. Capacity building in community health focuses on:

A) Reducing the skill levels of local healthcare providers.

B) Strengthening the community's ability to sustain health initiatives.

C) Isolating health initiatives from the influence of community needs.

D) Discouraging innovation and adaptation in health services.

9. **Community-based health planning is effective because it:**

A) Ignores the specific needs and contexts of the community.

B) Ensures interventions are culturally appropriate and targeted.

C) Focuses solely on the opinions of external experts.

D) Avoids engaging community members in the decision-making process.

10. **Adaptive capacity in health services refers to:**

A) The ability to provide the same services without change over time.

B) The resistance to adopting new technologies or methods.

C) The capability to adjust to emerging health threats and changing needs.

D) A focus on past successes without consideration for future challenges.

Answers:

1. B) Ensure long-term health benefits and resource conservation.

2. C) Adaptive capacity

3. C) Introducing new models or technologies to improve care.

4. C) Discouraging community participation in health planning

5. B) Adapting to changing health needs and priorities.

6. C) Improve access to care and the efficiency of health services.

7. C) Ensuring communities have resources for health infrastructure and services.

8. B) Strengthening the community's ability to sustain health initiatives.

9. B) Ensures interventions are culturally appropriate and targeted.

10. C) The capability to adjust to emerging health threats and changing needs.

Conclusion

The exploration of community health through this comprehensive journey has unveiled the multifaceted nature of health care delivery, public health policy, ethical considerations, and the pivotal role of sustainability and innovation in shaping healthier communities. From understanding the basics of community health, navigating health systems, and addressing ethical dilemmas, to embracing technological advancements and fostering resilience, this journey has highlighted the importance of integrated, community-centric approaches in public health.

The discussed chapters underscore the necessity of collaboration among healthcare providers, policymakers, community members, and other stakeholders to address the complex health challenges of today and tomorrow. Ethical considerations, particularly around confidentiality, consent, and community rights, serve as the foundation for trust and effective engagement in health initiatives. Meanwhile, sustainability and innovation are identified as key drivers for adapting health services to meet evolving needs and ensuring long-term health benefits for communities.

Fostering community resilience emerges as a critical strategy for preparing for and responding to health emergencies, underscoring the need for adaptable, resource-efficient, and culturally sensitive health initiatives. By building on the strengths of communities and leveraging advancements in health technology, public health efforts can achieve greater impact, ensuring equitable access to care and promoting the well-being of all community members.

In conclusion, the journey through community health reveals a dynamic field where continuous learning, ethical practice, and innovation are essential for advancing public health goals. As we move forward, the insights gained underscore the importance of a collective effort in building resilient, healthy, and sustainable communities for the future.

*The best way to thank an author is
to
write a review.*